New Book of Nutritional
and Medical Secrets

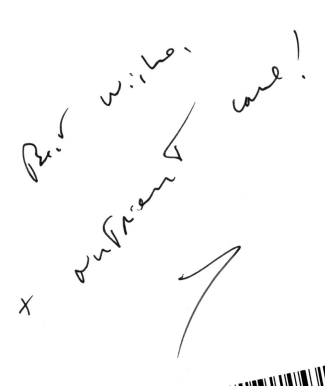

D1371981

New Book of Nutritional and Medical Secrets

Dr. David L. Vastola

ISBN-10: **1537684353**
ISBN 13: **9781537684352**

Contents

Introduction

F. Scott Fitzgerald said it best: "A secret is like being inside and outside at the same time." Perhaps that is why everyone likes a secret because it makes you, the keeper, very special. Within an instant, you become important, one of a kind, and desired by others for that very secret. The secrets that you are about to learn, however, about nutrients need to be shared for the welfare of yourself and others. That in and by itself will make you even more important.

In my first book, *Fountain of Youth: Making Sense of Vitamins, Minerals, Supplements, and Herbs*, I detail and review nutrients and briefly describe how they are used. In this second book, I intend to review the most common diseases, go over standard medical care, and then explain how nutrients can be *specifically* used. That's a well-kept secret—how to use nutrients correctly. The uses of nutrients, like medications, have certain commonalities, but they also have their differences, and these differences may be even more important. Just like the rules for using medications, the rules for using nutrients need to be adhered to, so knowing and understanding them is crucial. I will first discuss the general secrets and then delve into the more specific ones.

Let me ask you a question: Why are nutrients so important? It's a simple question but a really important one, since it is the basis for writing this book and can directly affect you and allow you to live longer and healthier. More than that, it should be an important part of your medical care, and a personalized one too. If that is all true—and it is true, I assure you—then what is the best way to get proper nutrients without being misled or deceived into trying regimens that are bogus? There are so many bogus ones that it is best to start from the beginning and develop an understanding of basic principles so as to remove any profit or political motives that could persuade you from the truth. These profit motives have different faces, but any time that you hear "vitamins," be on guard.

Recently, I had a drug representative in my office promoting a legitimate prescription drug. His assistance that his drug was better than his competitors' because his was combined with vitamins C and E; this tells you how important vitamins have become, because now they are market-driven and branded that way. By the way, when I mention vitamins, I mean vitamins only. There are minerals, trace elements, herbals, and other nutrients that need to be discussed in their proper framework, so get used to these differences. To be honest, it is you—the general public—that is driving the discussion and profit motive and is moving the research that is actively going on. Yes, there are universities that are making an honest attempt at researching vitamins, nutrients, and herbs. I'm grateful because that gives the research a certain amount of credibility.

Whatever the driving forces are, the use of vitamins is becoming a giant snowball that is gaining momentum down the hill of medical care. Even with all this going on, the vast medical community still does not recognize or want to recognize the importance of vitamins. Medical-school professors still don't provide for training in medical-school curricula about this topic; instead, they pawn it off to nutritionists. That's like shooting an elephant with a BB gun! Sorry, for me this lack of training is an insult, and because of the importance of vitamins, there should be a whole Department of Nutritional Studies in all our medical schools so the doctors taking care of you know about nutrients. Harvard, are you calling me?

In this book, I review research and define all the different types of nutrients—some good, some bad—but you will know the difference. By understanding the research, you will then be less likely to be fooled into buying something that is worthless. Research is not the same thing as naked claims, and it can be a marketing tool. Often terms such as *organic* or *natural* have no merit. Yes, because billions of dollars are being spent on vitamins and nutrients every year, marketers will try to fool you into thinking there may be benefit when in reality there likely is none. Since I can't hold all your hands while you are shopping, the next best thing is for me to provide you guidelines (secrets) to follow. I also define what *natural* and *organic* mean and attempt to put these terms in perspective.

What is exciting for me is that clinical studies are being done in large groups of patients who are taking *x* nutrient over *x* years—and these are the results as compared to a control group. At the same time, their basic chemistries are also being understood. As the body of laboratory data gets larger and larger, you can start to see a pattern that explains the critical nature of the research and gives real weight to evidence regarding why and how nutrients should be taken. As the studies stack up, one by one, eventually there will be other studies using them together, because of this cumulative approach it only makes sense. It's like treating high blood pressure with two to three different drugs to lower it through different mechanisms because just one will not always work effectively.

Over the past few years, the topic of aging has been reopened, and you can thank nutrients for that. Never before has the medical profession seriously bridged this subject, but people need to start asking themselves how they can slow down and even reverse the aging process. Nutrients, because of their intracellular (in the cell) activity, have opened this Pandora's box, and as part of eating properly and exercising, nutrients fit nicely.

Nutrients affect the most basic cell functions, such as renewal of the human cell after it wears out and performance of the cells' functions, such as thinking in the brain, pumping of the blood in the heart, or breathing in the lung. Nutrients also affect how cells perform these functions through cell energy by preserving mitochondrial function (structures in all cells that make energy for them to work) and by up-regulating (turning on good genes) and down-regulating genes (turning off bad genes).

The other exciting news about nutrients is that they can benefit many functions in our body at the same time. I read an article in the *Mayo Clinic Proceedings* that was titled "Vascular Remodeling," a direct offshoot of nutrient research, and that's part of the reason why nutrients are so difficult to categorize—because they are in so many places in our body at the same time. Think about it—cellular energy that will not wane with age and the protection of your cellular DNA. Wow, that's like the story of Methuselah, who lived to be 969 years of age. Finally, nutrients maintain our immune systems to avoid cancer and serious infections such as shingles that we develop as we get older.

In the book, I make reference to the BMI, which stands for body mass index—now the gold standard for obesity. It's a complicated formula, which is unimportant, but its significance *is* important. If your BMI is lower than 25, then you are not overweight. If it's 25–30, you are considered overweight, and if greater than 30, you are obese. There is one caveat, however. Someone who is muscular can have an increased BMI and not be overweight or obese, a fact that needs to be referenced in the person's medical chart so that insurance companies who have access to the charts don't label the person incorrectly, which could raise health insurance rates. That little important "gem" seems to get lost in the shuffle, so don't forget it, because the BMI is not the holy grail, as most people and insurance companies would like you to think. My intent is to give you a new understanding of how nutrients can help prevent and treat diseases like diabetes, heart disease, cancer, and Alzheimer's disease, but in the context of standard medical care. Together they are a potent force to keep you well and living longer. Ironically, with diseases like Alzheimer's disease, the nutrients seem to work better and are on the "front end" of helping the patients and their families deal with this dreadful disease.

One

Basic Secrets

_L_ ike building a house, building our body will only be as good as its foundation. These secrets therefore will be structured with this goal in mind, because as your health takes shape, the more healthy you will become.

I start out with some small, general secrets in order to not overwhelm you, but I can promise that there will be a crescendo toward the larger ones. I apologize that there will be some repetition, but that is the nature of the beast (nutritional therapies) because there is a lot of overlap. Also, the repetition especially of the mechanisms and physiology will only reinforce the how, why, and when to use them, thus eliminating memorization.

The first secret is to specifically tailor the nutrient to the problem. It's like digitalis, which is effective for patients who have congestive heart failure but not for everyone. There are a few exceptions, which I will categorize as antiaging or general medical care (GMC), but, by and large, this book provides you with a logical, medically oriented approach (an outline) on how to tailor the nutrient to the problem. The provided research for each nutrient will then give you the rationale for why I recommend something. It's a fundamental premise in medicine to tailor drug therapies, and the same is true of nutrients. Look at it this way—if I lined up a hundred patients on nutrients, they would all be taking different combinations. In my review of each nutrient, I also outline the medical diseases involved and explain how they would present with symptoms. Therefore, you will have an opportunity, by reading this book, to go to a mini–medical school.

The second secret in using nutrients is what I call perpetuity, which means that they have to be taken over a long period of time to be effective. Medications, however, like antibiotics, will have a measured effect within hours and last only for short periods of time (days or weeks). Nay, not so with nutrients. The reason for this is that nutrients depend on micro tissue (cell) levels, which may take weeks or months to achieve. Drugs, on the other hand, are taken in mega cellular doses; therefore, their effect will be much quicker. This secret is important to remember because, in my experience, it's hard for patients to take anything and spend their money for a long time when they are feeling well.

Finally, "effects" such as living longer may take many decades to appreciate. People are becoming more health conscious, but unfortunately are distracted by things such as organic food and a workout that includes only "looking good" or the "peacock phenomenon," when in fact neither will do anything for their health. Hopefully, this book will dispel that nonsense and give to you, the reader, who is legitimately interested, a path to a longer and healthier life. Those organic turnips will not save your life! Since organic "anything" has not been shown to increase life span.

The third secret in taking nutrients is that they have to be considered in the context of each patient. Some considerations include the following: What does that mean? What is the gender of the patient? Age? Size? Costs? Other medical conditions and other medications that he or she is taking? This total context will determine what nutrient or nutrients would be appropriate and how much, which can be daunting and not easy to determine. If prescribing nutrients were that easy, everyone would be doing it. There is this pervasive notion out there, however, that nutrients are minor league, but this belief couldn't be further from the truth. We must remember that standard medications are also prescribed in this manner, and there is no difference.

Finally, with new revelations through blood tests about BNP (beta natiuro-peptide) and galectin—which provide early indications of heart disease—nutrients such as lipoic acid, carnitine, and branched-chain amino acids are indicated even if patient feels well and without symptoms. That should stir even the greatest of nutrient skeptics and seed the interest for others, because as miraculous as it sounds, nutrients can reverse heart disease. Also, words such as *mitochondria* and *NFkB,* which are related to aging and cancer can point to possible problems even when the patient presents with no symptoms. This all make sense in the arena of nutrients. Exciting, isn't it?

The fourth secret has to do with purchasing your nutrients. Since the FDA does not control them, do not buy the cheapest, because you will not know what you are getting. It's that simple! One study that analyzed the content of krill oil, for example, found that many commercial brands had very low or no krill oil in them at all. All the brands that I recommend have been analyzed for content, and I know that when my patients use them, they are getting what they are supposed to get.

How can you determine if something is working or not working if you don't know what you are taking? Another good example is the cheap DHEA that will only work in rats because humans lack the enzyme to convert it. Many times, patients will shop around for the cheapest brands and end up getting very little of the active ingredient, which won't work unless you're a rat!

The fifth secret with nutrients is that often they have to be taken in combination with other nutrients. Of course, that brings up the whole subject of when and how to take multiple nutrients, because that practice can consume your whole day. This is a good point to introduce a new concept that I call grazing. It means what it says: take a small amount of the nutrients all day long (spread them out), knowing that you can take them together.

The sixth secret is where to store your nutrients. Storing your nutrients really falls within the same domain as storing your medications, so keep them in a cool, dry room and make sure to check the expiration dates. Therefore, the hot and humid bathroom is not where to store them. I would keep them along with your standard medications in the kitchen, and that way, you won't lose them or forget to take them. Do not worry, the heat from the kitchen has not been shown to degrade nutrients.

The seventh secret is not to underestimate their effects, benefits, or potential undesired side effects. A day doesn't go by that I'm not discontinuing or decreasing the dose of nutrients that my patients take because of undesirable side effects. Even the medical community doesn't appreciate their benefit or potential for harm. For example, before surgery, doctors will tell patients to stop *all* nutrients because doctors do not know how the nutrients will affect the surgery.

The eighth secret is to take them. I tell patients to keep them with their medications so as not to forget, or put them in an obvious place, like on the kitchen counter, especially if they are taking them slowly over the course of a day (grazing). Believe it or not, common sense does come into play. It's been shown that to be successful in your daily routines, such as finding car keys or performing other tasks, you must develop a routine for where you put them, at a certain time of day, and so forth.

In summary, these initial secrets really do put you on the inside and outside at the same time. They will be your holy grail to a longer life, which was the green light that Gatsby followed.

Two

THE SECRETS OF UNDERSTANDING MEDICAL PROBLEMS

*I*n order to understand the specifics of nutritional therapies, you will need to understand the basics of medical care. Health-care professionals never discuss these principles with the general public, because they are so general and non-specific that they are lost in the shuffle, but I'm convinced that once you know them, your overall health care will get better.

One of the greatest secrets in life and in this book is to use common sense, which is nothing more than an extension of the dictum of Occam's razor, which tells us that the simplest explanation is generally the correct one.

In order to understand my commonsense and concise approach to medicine, we need to first have a framework and background about medical information to build on. In the process, I will develop the nomenclature for you to speak the language of medicine and gain an understanding of the medical problems that affect us. Building on that, you will know why particular symptoms are relevant and what exactly is occurring, so, finally, you will gain the knowledge about medication and treatment (nutritional) programs to avoid needless mistakes.

The body is a highly complicated, integrated system, which is interconnected by various life-sustaining mechanisms. It is like a building with various apartments in it, but each apartment is a vital area that needs to be interconnected or integrated for the building to function normally and to survive. If the body functions normally, the apartment building (your body) is then in what is known as a homeostatic or healthy state. In contrast, a disease simply is a malfunction of one of these apartments, which may disrupt other apartments that then disrupt homeostatic function. So let's go through a brief summary of some of these systems, or apartments, to understand better how the body works.

Let's start with the heart. It's a good place to start, since heart disease is the most common disease found in the United States and the most common cause of death. For example, cardiovascular death accounts for almost a third of all deaths in men and women in the United States today. The cardiovascular system is just what it says: your heart and blood vessels, including both arteries and veins.

The heart (one apartment) is a pump, pumping blood to the rest of your body, with the arteries or highways carrying the blood out into other apartments to nourish them, and then the veins bring the blood back to your lungs to become oxygenated—and then the cycle repeats itself.

Dysfunction of the cardiovascular system affects the distribution of blood into all the organ systems, or apartments, or disrupts return of blood to the lungs for oxygenation, which therefore can affect the entire building. Knowing and understanding that concept is critical since it is the *main transport* system of nutrients, or vital services to the apartment complex, and also the main waste-removal service.

Your heart is nourished by coronary arteries, not by the blood inside it, and these arteries come off the aortic, or main, artery leaving your heart. Atherosclerosis, or hardening of these arteries, will cause heart dysfunction and a plethora of medical problems: angina, lowered pumping efficiency (congestive heart failure), arrhythmia (abnormal rhythm), and others. Finally, the heart works automatically through its own nervous system—its batteries are included, so to speak. These are the intrinsic pacemakers, and any dysfunction in this area leads to arrhythmia, or abnormal heartbeat.

If the venous system becomes dysfunctional, mainly through dilated veins, then fluid leaks out into the tissue, mainly into the legs. This in turn causes edema, or swelling, that results in a decreased venous return to the heart, which will decrease much-needed oxygen for the rest of the apartments.

Obviously, I should discuss your lungs next, and the secret is that they are closely linked and interconnected with your heart. Your lungs receive blood directly from your heart apartment. Their primary function is to oxygenate it by taking oxygen out of the air that you breathe and exchanging it for carbon dioxide, a waste product, out of your blood, which interchanges which exchanges one carbon dioxide molecule for one oxygen molecule, one molecule for one molecule. Therefore, your lungs are nothing more than an exchange system for oxygenating your blood and removing the waste product, carbon dioxide.

This is important because the lungs are so interrelated to cardiovascular dynamics through the pulmonary arterial/venous circulation system that any cardiac dysfunction will also negatively impact lung function and vice versa. For example, congestive heart failure (CHF) results in decreased oxygen and shortness of breath, while COPD (chronic obstructive pulmonary disease) can lead to heart failure. Therefore, it is not uncommon to have patients who have both cardiovascular problems and related pulmonary disease. There you have it: another part of this integrated system, or apartment complex, affecting another.

The digestive system—which is near and dear to me because I'm a gastroenterologist—does just what it says: it digests food. This system includes your esophagus, stomach, pancreas, small and large intestines, and liver and has to do with the absorption and processing of food substrates. The secret here is that your gastrointestinal (GI) tract is *not* part of your body, but a tunnel going through it. That's right; it's *outside* your body, like an elevator shaft within the apartment complex, and it has no contact with your body's actual metabolic function or apartments.

The GI tract needs the stomach, the bile from the liver, enzymes from the pancreas, and absorption through the small intestine, however, to accomplish this, since the food, in order to be absorbed, has to be processed (broken down) first. Once broken down, food is then taken to the appropriate apartments, where the elevator door opens and the food exits to do its thing (be reassembled).

Your colon is a storage organ where no absorption occurs. Therefore, your GI apartment separates out various food substrates, breaks them down, absorbs what is wanted, and then excretes what isn't wanted, like garbage from the

7

apartment complex. Your colon then becomes the "solid waste authority," by storing waste until it is picked up or excreted (no recycling bins included!).

The endocrine system is a system of hormones. Hormones are defined as chemical substances that are released directly into your bloodstream to other tissues or apartments, where they are taken up by receptors to do their needed effects. You have heard of some of these hormones: cortisone, insulin, thyroid, and estrogen. These are hormones that are important for sustaining your blood pressure, controlling blood sugars, and performing many other metabolic functions, but there are also many, many other endocrine glands, which are like little subset apartments in this giant apartment complex. The glands keep all the engineering services of the apartment complex integrated and working (for example, they keep the lights on, control the heat and temperature, provide sleep and rest, and, last but not least, maintain reproductive function). They function as general service items in the apartment building—with, I guess, the reproductive ones being the game room or family room!

It's not such a great secret that the brain is a giant computer that sits on top of your body, evaluating everything that is going on from sensory impulses, making decisions for you, and then carrying out your activities through its motor system. It does so through a wiring system called the spinal cord that comes out of the back of the brain, with wires going out into your extremities and other organ parts. The brain also receives impulses—called sensory input—from body parts to know what's going on. Without these electrical connections from the body to the brain, and vice versa, the brain would have no way of knowing what was affecting it and how to carry out appropriate responses.

A large part of this sensory input also comes from hearing, smelling, touching, feeling pain, and seeing. The decision-making process is the reason that we are able to adapt and survive, and, as you can well imagine, a lot of wiring is required, both central and peripheral, which therefore can become vulnerable to trauma and other diseases. Without this master computer, the apartment would not be coordinated in an organized fashion, and chaos would result.

Your musculoskeletal system is a system of muscles, joints, and bones that are your support and transport systems: your mainframe. The secret is this: the musculoskeletal system is one of the few areas that is not well appreciated by the medical profession (your doctor). It functions through physical strength and joint performance but still depends on all other apartments or systems to work properly. For example, if either your cardiovascular apartment, which supplies nutrients to your muscles, or your nervous system, which supplies the coordination through wiring (your nerves), becomes dysfunctional, then you won't move as well as you should. As you can see, one system affects the other because they are integrated and depend on each other.

Your liver apartment has something like 160 metabolic functions, many of which detoxify and excrete things from your blood. It changes these impurities chemically and discharges them out through the bile into the gallbladder for storage, and finally excretes them out your GI tract. The liver also manufactures protein-clotting factors to prevent bleeding; bile to digest fat; and glutathione, which is one of the body's strongest antioxidants.

The liver is also a massive storage organ for things like sugar and vitamin B12. For example, it has enough vitamin B12 to last four to five years with no intake, so the secret here is that vegetarians who do not get B12 (through meat) will not experience any problems with the deficiency for four to five years. In summary, within the liver apartment, the renal-liver complex functions to maintain homeostasis through waste removal, and the liver also produces necessities needed by the apartment complex.

Last but not least are your kidneys. We have two kidneys, but, rarely, some people congenitally have only one kidney, and this apartment is responsible for the filtration of the substances in the blood that are of no use and could be toxic. As substances flow through the kidney-filtration system, the body takes back what is important and necessary and, at the same time, releases what you don't need in the urine. This process is done via the GFR (glomerular filtration rate), which we can measure with blood flow through the kidney.

In addition, the kidneys are also indirectly related to high blood pressure since about 5 percent of all patients who have high blood pressure have kidney problems that can arise from insufficient blood flow to the kidneys. That causes an elevation of a substance called renin from the kidneys, which will increase blood pressure. Finally, your kidney apartment helps maintain pH and electrolyte balance.

This is a brief survey of your body's integrated systems, and I would hope that you can now understand how complicated your body must be in order to maintain homeostatic function and stay healthy. If one of these systems, or one of the apartments in the apartment complex, does not work, it can directly and indirectly affect many of the others. The secret is that this integration of *interrelated* systems (apartments) explains human disease.

Without much imagination, you can also see how medications can either help or screw things up, and how they are excreted can also be vitally important, because if medications are under excreted, they can make you toxic. When a patient comes to my office with a particular complaint, therefore, my job is to see which one of these apartments is not functioning correctly, along with how substances and drugs may be excreted. Knowing that, I can identify what diseases might be affecting the patient, and I can clearly determine treatment.

Let me give an example. Let's say you develop an infection and come in complaining of a cough. You're bringing up yellow sputum and have fever and chills with shortness of breath. By history, in going through all these symptoms, I determine that you may have dysfunction of your lung apartment system. On physical examination, I can hear things in your lungs, which is consistent with the symptoms. By the nature of your symptoms—age, type of onset, smoking history, and physical findings, for example—I can determine then that you have a bacterial infection of your lungs and then treat you with appropriate medications and antibiotics. Of course, the actual treatment is a bit more complicated, but this basic protocol is how it works along with the application of nutrients.

One of the most basic concepts of nutrient treatments is oxidation. Caused by many things and also because of the day-to-day consequences of being alive, free radicals are formed when the process of using oxygen in the body creates a chemical reaction that causes the loss of an outer-ring electron from an atom. Thus a free radical is formed. These free radicals are stressful to our cells. Unless neutralized with antioxidants (electron donors), the cell will become dysfunctional and may even become cancerous over time. In summary, by stealing electrons from other molecules (oxidation), any of the apartments that I've talked about can be affected.

Another secret here is that common sense would suggest that by giving patients enough antioxidants with electron donors, we could prevent excessive oxidation from these free radicals and therefore prevent disease. As an extension of this thesis, this theory runs over into the aging process itself, with the belief that these same free radicals cause aging. I think that this is probably partially true, since it makes sense, but there are other factors for the aging process (for more details, see the section on "General Medical Care" in chapter 19).

Let's go back to our previous example of the patient with a lung infection. This patient obviously came in contact with the bacterium that caused inflammation in the lungs and the pneumonia that caused the signs and symptoms that the patient was having. As mentioned, it was believed by the medical community that this is all done through the single chemical process of oxidation, so if this same patient had sustained himself or herself with high amounts of antioxidants, the problem could have theoretically been prevented or decreased in severity, even if the patient had been subjected to this same bacterium. This premise of mine is a very far-reaching one and even now touches on the aging process itself.

Finally, aging has been accepted more or less as a fait accompli (it will happen no matter what we do). When I first started practicing medicine thirty years ago, it was unheard of to perform surgery on patients in their seventies and eighties because the risk was too great, but now we operate on people in their eighties and nineties. Despite their far-advanced heart disease and through complicated procedures, the overall mortality and morbidity rates for older patients are good. Therefore, aging from a medical standpoint has become relative and moot because people are living much longer.

It has been estimated by aging experts (Dr. Aubrey deGrey at Cambridge University) that our bodies have been engineered to live about 150 years. This sounds almost Orwellian or futuristic, but understanding more about the genetics of disease, antioxidants, and a plethora of new medications and discoveries that occur almost on a weekly basis could make this possible. This concept is important for all of us, even the healthy ones, because it should get our attention and change our focus to prevention—not just to the reactive treatment of disease.

Health is more than repairing this apartment complex; it is making sure it doesn't run down and get sick because of the lack of maintenance. Ironically, most people take better care of their cars and boats than of their own bodies, which should be a wake-up call. Why? Ridding any disease process that can take you out, maintaining normal function of the apartment, and preventing any potential problem for the apartments is a strategy that I emphasize to my patients. It is also cheaper by keeping you out of the hospital and ER.

Three

The Secrets of Illnesses

*I*t sounds simple, but you would be surprised how many doctors don't even realize when you are sick. It is a fundamental axiom in medicine for the doctor to know that and separate illnesses from any of the social stresses that all of us are being confronted with every day, and then for the doctor to recommend an appropriate regimen for treatment, including nutrients.

For the doctor, illnesses are really a dilemma that presents in two dimensions. The first dimension is this: Are you sick or not sick? The second dimension is this: If you are truly sick, what is causing it? So let's deal with the questions in that order.

When I was working at the Meyer Memorial Hospital in Buffalo, New York and Cook County Hospital in Chicago, both of which are huge hospitals with large emergency rooms and over a thousand beds each, it became obvious to me that one of the most important questions that needed to be answered before a proper diagnosis and treatment could be established was this: Is this patient sick? It sounds trivial and easy, but it is probably one of the most profound questions there is in regard to taking care of patients.

In a large emergency room, you can watch the medical team's approach to patients, and within a short period of time, you can sort out who will become the best doctors on the basis of their ability to identify who is sick and who is not sick. The secret is that those doctors who can triage (sort out) effectively have won half the battle.

Basically, true illnesses, or disruptions of these apartments (the various organ systems in the body), depend on the severity of the problem (symptoms) and also duration of the symptoms. We can have minor symptoms for many, many years, and they will remain unimportant and seem normal because they have withstood the test of time. After a while, the symptoms become a normal way of life. If these symptoms were important, you would be dead. Many times, however, if these long-term problems change character, they then will need medical investigation.

For example, if you have constipation, and you are only going to the bathroom every two to three days, and that now becomes four to five days, then the change needs to be investigated. If you develop a new problem that lasts longer than three to five days, then probably you should seek medical attention, but if your issue involves severe pain and/or bleeding, then immediate attention is necessary. Therefore, the first part is for you to decide whether you are sick or not and, depending on the facts that I have just outlined, decide when to seek medical attention and what to do about it. In summary, ask yourself, "Is one of my apartments in trouble, and do I need a repair person?"

The standard approach that physicians use is to take a personal history and family history, followed by a physical examination with laboratory confirmation. The secret here is that it is vitally important that a detailed history be taken and that it should include not only the current problem, but also the personal (smoking, alcohol), medications, family, and past medical history, because the history in its entirety will generally make a diagnosis about 85 percent of the time, even without a physical or laboratory confirmation. If your doctor spends a limited amount of time with your history, then a diagnosis will be difficult, if not impossible, to achieve, so my advice is to go elsewhere if this occurs.

The physical examination occurs next and should be relevant not only to the complaints, but also to other related organs, or apartments. For example, if you are complaining of chest pains, your doctor should take your blood pressure and check your heart, weight, temperature, lungs, abdomen, and all other related organs, or apartments. The reason for doing this is that since the apartments are integrated (connected), there may be clues or evidence in other areas of your body that will lead to a diagnosis.

For example, the chest pain may be more easily diagnosed with a rectal exam and a positive stool sample for blood. How so? Esophagitis, or an atypical gastric ulcer with bleeding, can cause chest pain—it's all integrated! This condition occurs because the slow bleeding results in an anemia that decreases the oxygen supplied to the heart, thus causing angina. Also, there may be the possibility of two or three other problems going on simultaneously. Therefore, the secret is that following the history, a complete physical examination of all the apartments needs to be done. That is one of the problems with subspecialties in this country today. These specialists only do their thing in "their" apartment and disregard the rest of the apartments, which makes a diagnosis very difficult. Then the patient will require multiple doctors instead of just one, which is a lot more expensive, and disjointed care can be very inefficient.

The secret with the laboratory is that the laboratory is nothing more than a way of confirming what the doctor thinks is going on. All too frequently, doctors will use the laboratories and x-rays to make a diagnosis, only to find themselves in a quagmire of not knowing exactly what is going on because of lab and x-ray variations. Frequently, these exams contradict themselves and give you a false positive or a false negative result, making a correct diagnosis even harder.

There is nothing worse than a missed diagnosis, which then leads to a wrong treatment plan and a waste of time and money—and even death. I have seen, time and time again, physicians making erroneous diagnoses because they relied too heavily on the lab and x-rays. So remember, the secret is that the history and physical are more important than the lab and x-ray results, which should only be used to confirm the diagnosis, not the reverse.

Theoretically, at this stage, when it has been decided that you are sick and the doctor has examined you, then a diagnosis needs to be made and treatment begun. Depending on the nature of the problem and number of apartments involved, along with how ill-defined the disease may be, it may take several visits and more advanced testing to make a diagnosis. This could involve sophisticated studies like CT scans, MRIs, special blood tests, endoscopies, and even further consultation with other physicians who are experts in the other apartments.

It is very big secret and is vitally important that a diagnosis, *the root cause*, be achieved, because then you can answer all the questions that might follow (such as treatment, cost, contagiousness, and prognosis). Don't treat symptoms. Treat the root cause, because you don't want to treat a patient having a heart attack with only pain medication!

Another secret that can help you and your doctor in making a diagnosis is to relate symptoms to an organ system or apartment. For example, if you have abdominal pain, when does it hurt? ("It hurts when I eat, and it gets worse.") For another example, let's talk about chest pain. If you are having chest pain, you need to ask yourself what organ systems, or apartments, are in your chest. The major apartment systems within the chest include your heart, esophagus, and lungs. There are other things in the chest that can cause pain, but these are the major ones that would account for almost 90–95 percent of all illnesses with chest pain, so that is where you need to concentrate your efforts.

Ask yourself, "What makes the pain better or what makes it worse?" In doing so, you can often differentiate it. Like your apartment, if it's worse when you turn the lights on, then it must be an electrical problem. If the pain you are having in your chest is made worse when you eat or gets better when you eat, then you know it is probably associated with your gastrointestinal apartment—the esophagus or stomach. If the pain you are having in your chest is worse when you breathe, then probably it is related to your pulmonary/lung apartment. Finally, if the chest pain is worse when you exert yourself and gets better when you rest, then it's most likely coming from your heart apartment.

Pain and bleeding deserve less discussion because most patients who have them would seek medical care immediately, unless the person is an idiot (no secret here). If pain and bleeding are not severe or massive, I would avoid the emergency room, since you will spend many, many hours there and achieve very little other than getting a big bill. The ER docs will ultimately refer you back to your private doctor anyway. The ERs are geared for true emergencies; they are not diagnostic centers. That is why it is so important to have your own doctor who knows you the best, so you can call him or her first and be seen quickly. In addition, if the ER is necessary, your doctor will call there to give the ER staff all the medical information they would need to expedite your treatment, thus saving time.

Finally, make sure that there are no delays to the management of the problem, and try to assist your doctor by being prepared to answer these types of questions prior to seeing him or her. Write your questions down beforehand, if necessary, and bring them with you to help you remember. Providing a good, accurate history and finding the relationship that we mentioned for organ apartment systems will make an easier job for your doctor and also increase the success rate. In addition, bring a list of all your medications, doses, and nutrients that you are taking. Don't fib or underplay about drinking, smoking, or drug use; be honest, since these will affect all the apartments, and their use is critical in understanding the nature of your problem.

Four

THE SECRETS OF A HEALTH STRATEGY FOR DIET AND EXERCISE

Like constructing a strong building, your health will depend on its foundation, and the basics will determine your ultimate future, which leads me to diet and exercise. "Diet and exercise" sounds easy, but with so much conflicting misinformation, it gets lost in the shuffle.

It's an axiomatic secret in medicine that diet and exercise are a must. Whether you're twenty, forty, sixty, or ninety years old, the formula for longevity and good health begins with diet and exercise. In addition, regardless of whatever disease you're talking about and the complexity of your treatment plan, the secret to a successful treatment will also require a good diet and exercise.

How can such a simple concept be so true? The reason is that we must return to the basics and leave out the confusion, conjecture, and rush to science and profiteering by other influences in the marketplace that abound and are manifested by the Internet (the information "toilet") and television. When you go to a bookstore, say Barnes and Noble, and look for an appropriate book to guide you in either diet or exercise, you find a shelf full of many different types of books describing all different types of plans that have their own unique answers to this problem. What this tells you, of course, is that no one has the answer (until now), which is very confusing!

Diet

Diet is a simple balance among calories taken in, your nutrient needs, and calories worked off—and also, I think, the need for vitamin, mineral, and antioxidant supplementation. I don't think that through our diets we can get the amount of antioxidants we need to maintain and to fend off the scourge of many diseases including aging, so they have to be supplemented. Therefore, the secret here is that we need supplements, which are inexpensive, relevant to our individual needs, and prudent, but that we also need to avoid shot gunning them. Look at it this way—the apartments need this "formula" to stay "livable."

Let me interrupt myself to tell you an interesting story. We have three toy poodles, and our oldest, when we bought her, was an apricot color, though her fur eventually turned white. Over the last two to three months, she started to convert back to the apricot color, so I took her a veterinarian. He said that her color change was due to her aging, and it is not unusual and nothing could be done. Well, what I did was put her on a good "doggie" multivitamin. Within two months, her apricot color had disappeared. She is now all white again, with a new sense of life. I realize this is only an anecdote—just one personal story— but it has merit and may be extrapolated to our own lives. As a matter of fact, I am sure it does!

If you are a woman, you should maintain your calorie input at about 2,000 calories per day, and for men, 3,000 calories per day, but the secret is that this is hard to do and of course depends on just how active you are. Marines, for example, will easily work off 10,000–12,000 calories per day, and that needs to calculate in. Simply cutting out fats and fried foods and decreasing portion size by a third will decrease calorie count by 50 percent. The Japanese do it, and look at them!

Also, studies comparing diets have been done many times, and the winner in respect to amount of weight loss, over the short and long terms, along with normalization of blood work (that is, lowering of lipids), is the Dr. Atkins diet. Yes, the high-fat diet is the best because the real culprit is not fat, but sugar and carbohydrates, which cause insulin surges along with cancer because insulin is also a growth factor. In a recent *Time* magazine article by Bryan Walsh called

"Eat Butter," Walsh reviewed all the new data and arrived at the same conclusion as Dr. Atkins did and that yours truly did as well. The medical profession was wrong, dead wrong, all these years because the doctors advised telling patients to not eat saturated fats but that carbohydrates were OK. More recently, it has been discovered that the sugar industry may have paid off a few Harvard professors to say publically that very thing.

The second best diet is the Mediterranean diet, which is my choice (I'm Italian, surprise!), which I will institute after the desired weight loss is achieved using the Atkins diet. The short-term and long-term labs are also very good with this diet, so there is some validity to my choice other than my Italian roots, but the converse is also true. If you are too thin, you will also have a decreased life expectancy because of the cellular stress that low weight causes, so being too skinny is not good either.

My plan, therefore, with overweight patients is to start with the Atkins diet. Once the patient has attained his or her ideal body mass index (BMI of 25–30), then I switch him or her over to the Mediterranean diet. So the true secret here is the blend of the Mediterranean and Atkins diets over a long period of time. You need to view this diet plan as a general service-maintenance contract for your apartments to keep them running smoothly, like your heating and cooling systems. There is nothing worse than having your heat go out in the winter up north, or your air conditioning fail in the summer (especially in Florida).

Another aspect with this exercise model is when to do it. Patients are constantly trying to find time to exercise, especially with their busy lives. The Japanese for years have incorporated exercise into work. In the movie *Gung Ho* with Michael Keaton, this Japanese car company does that very thing by incorporating exercise into their workers' lives. At lunchtime, which they are paid for, workers exercise. For me, this is a great idea since, if I wait until after work, I'm too tired to do it, so I do it before work, although having to get up so early is not easy.

Here's another interesting aspect for the employer. A University of Bristol study reported that lunchtime exercise, including aerobics and stretching, increased management skills by 28 percent, productivity by 17 percent, and mental and interpersonal performance by 11 percent. In addition, there were fewer sick days, a decrease in obesity, and decreased insurance costs. The secret of incorporating exercise and work helped both the business and the employee, which is a huge twofer (two for one).

Let me give you an example. In my first book, *Fountain of Youth: Making Sense of Vitamins, Minerals, Supplements, and Herbs* (to be published by Carrel Books), I go into a lot of detail about what the oils do and how they work. The omega-3 oils and olive oil (extra virgin) should be taken every day, because they decrease overall cholesterol levels; increase HDL; and, finally, decrease atherogenesis, which has been shown in both animal and human studies in addition to producing many other benefits. Also, it has been shown that patients who take the oils and who have bypass surgery have a closure (how long the artery stays open) of about 30 percent less. Their anti-inflammatory resolution molecules make these oils useful in arthritis and for colitis patients (those with ulcerative and Crohn's disease) by decreasing inflammation. Basically, the oils keep your apartments functioning by decreasing the organic "rust" in your metabolic engines.

A good multivitamin regimen needs to be considered if you are intensively dieting or are underweight, so that you get trace elements, since most brand multivitamins have nothing else of benefit. Each nutrient needs absolute *amounts* of what is required, not the RDA (recommended daily allowance), which is out dated and useless. For example, the RDA for vitamin C is 60 mg per day, (that is set by government doctors) when in reality it is 2,000 mg per day for women and 3,000 mg per day for men.

Let me give you an example of how you need to look at nutrients. The recommended daily allowance (RDA) of vitamin E is 15 international units (IU), but, in actuality, you need 200–800 IU of vitamin E. If you had the proper amount of all the vitamins in a multivitamin, it would be the size of a Volkswagen. Furthermore, I would recommend that you do not take synthetic vitamin E, since it is the only vitamin that has poor absorption; you can tell whether it is synthetic by reading the label. If it says "dL tocopherol," it is synthetic and not good, whereas "d tocopherol" is natural and therefore the one to buy.

More recently, it has been shown that alpha and gamma isomers of tocopherol are best to help lower heart disease, so look for them on the label, which would say "alpha and gamma d tocopherol." It matters less whether all other vitamins are synthetic or not, so you can take the synthetic ones, which are cheaper and save you money.

Another example is vitamin C, which, in my estimation, should be taken while dieting in quantities of at least 2,000 mg per day for all women and 3,000 mg per day for all men every day. Dr. Linus Pauling, who won two Nobel Prizes in chemistry, recommended taking vitamin C in doses of 8,000–10,000 mg a day, and everyone thought that he was crazy. Guess what? He was right to some extent.

At my recommended doses (just shared with you on the prior page), vitamin C increases immunity; stops skin hemorrhaging; improves cardiovascular function, especially during stressful situations; and helps the body during stress or allergic scenarios. Finally, like vitamins C and E, and with the omega-3 oils, many more nutrients need to be tailored to the individual problems and the patient's needs along with their appropriate doses.

Exercise

I would be remiss if I didn't talk about exercise. You will also find at the bookstore and on the Internet many types of exercise plans, with various gurus and other experts trying to espouse exercise programs that will benefit you. Does Richard Simmons sound familiar? Every celebrity on the planet has the right answer! I'm not sure whether they all really believe what they are advising or if they are just trying to sell their books—probably both—but I'm reminded, and you should be too, of how the cardiac exercise programs were devised.

In the 1980s, Dr. Barnard Lown at Harvard University studied John Havlicek, who was a professional basketball player for the Boston Celtics, because of his physical stamina and endurance. Havlicek could run up and down the basketball court full speed for hours on end without any dramatic drop in his basketball performance. When they studied him at Harvard, they found that the ejection fraction from his heart—the amount of blood pumped out with each contraction—was anywhere from three to four times what you would find in a normal person. As a result, his heart did not have to work as hard to fulfill his exercise needs; therefore, he could last longer and do more.

You see, the secret here is that the fundamental equation for cardiac (heart) function is cardiac output (CO) = stroke volume (SV) × heart rate (HR). Simply put, your blood volume coming out of your heart will increase if either or both the SV and HR increase, and will commensurately decrease if either or both go down.

John Havlicek's CO (cardiac output) was three to four times greater than normal, thereby allowing his HR (heart rate) to be much lower and conserving energy to go much further. In other words, his heart was so strong that it conserved energy to be used later to increase his endurance.

More studies found that in order for normal people like you to do this, it will require three hours a week of a sustained, elevated heart rate (isometrics), which can be done very nicely with power walking. That's all. Just three hours a week, and no running or jogging is required. In my humble opinion, running should not be done to maintain your healthy ways because it will eventually ruin your joints. When compared, running and power walking have equal benefit. Also, running will increase the free radical pool in your lungs, which over time damages the lungs with fibrosis (scarring).

This concept of sustaining any muscle is called isometrics and will in time strengthen it, and the *sustaining* aspect is what is key. In summary, using these cardiovascular "apartment" isometrics, your heart will remain strong and, if it is stronger, will be less likely to get diseased. You will be able to do more and remain healthy. Even if you develop, for example, coronary artery disease, you will have the strength and reserve to survive.

These studies were conclusive for me and have been useful guidelines that I use with recommendations for my patients with all types of heart disease. Simply put, all you need to do for exercise to maintain health and also prevent disease is three hours weekly of semi-strenuous activity to generate an increased, sustained heart rate. Heart function will improve and be maintained, and the circulation to all your apartments will be provided for.

Besides heart isometrics, I believe that lifting weights for your upper and lower body is a must to maintain your strength and also to help burn calories.

The secret here is that muscles burn calories in and by themselves, which can add up to about 200–300 calories a day, which is a freebie, and will also allow you to be more physical (through tennis or playing golf, for example) and work off more calories. This is a positive cycle. As you get older, you will realize that most cycles are the negative ones, which is the reality of aging and getting old.

The third part of this holy trinity of exercise is stretching. As we get older, we become less flexible and stiffer because our support tissues begin to retract. The muscles, tendons, and support tissues like collagen are all included. You have seen professional athletes stretch before they compete, and they do it to become better equipped to use their musculoskeletal system for whatever they do. There is evidence also to suggest that if you are more nimble and less stiff, you are less likely to get injured.

The secret here, and a corollary to this with stiffness, is imbalance. We become unstable, making it more probable that we can fall, which can result in hip and other fractures. Therefore, I recommend that yoga or tai chi be added to your exercise program. In doing so, the aforementioned balance and stiffness problems improve dramatically. Twice weekly is enough, and forget about that hot yoga, which has no physiological basis and only subjects you to the risks of hyperthermia and hypotension. One last thing: if you think that yoga is a piece of cake, think again. It is hard, really hard, and despite its obvious benefits, you will not be looking forward to going. I didn't!

As an addendum, a very useful secret is to try to do your exercise with your spouse, friends, or neighbors—like adjoining apartments, a form of group therapy—because other people can help initiate your practice, and then you will more likely do it. For example, my wife and I exercise together, but there are times when both of us are tired. Yet a phone call from our exercise "buddies," nudging us to go along with them, gets us out there, whereas otherwise we would not have gone.

Another secret in regard to time spent exercising, especially if there are time limitations, is that exercise can be broken up into ten-minute sessions that have the same value as doing it all at once. For example, three ten-minute sessions are just as good for you as one thirty-minute session.

For some reason, we have this common belief that you have to exercise for one hour, or otherwise you won't benefit from it. The other aspect and secret of exercise is weight resistance. When lifting weights, you need to do twelve to fifteen repetitions with three sets. Doing this will maximize muscle strengthening and guarantee endurance to help support metabolic function. You see, this apartment is really the mainframe or superstructure for all the rest, so it's vitally important.

In summary, if you're not on a proper diet and exercise program, your apartment complex is at risk for malfunction where human disease, as we define it, occurs. Remember, maintaining your homeostasis (the normal state of the apartments) in the long term cannot be done with medication alone, and you know what happens when the foundation is not supportive anymore: the apartments can become permanently weakened. Ironically, I take care of a few ship captains who command huge yachts, and they take better care of their boat engines than their own bodies' metabolic engines. Explain that to me. You, however, as the captain of your yacht (your body), should make sure that you do not do the same thing.

Five

TREATMENT SECRETS

Treatments come in many different forms and not just as medications. Granted, medications are the lion's share, but the true art of medicine is the dispensing of the total picture, including nutrients. Knowing what to do and how to navigate the medical system requires much learning for the doctor, coupled with the savvy of common sense with caring.

The next step is that if you are sick, with an established diagnosis, one of the apartments is not working well, so how do you know that the treatment you are receiving is proper?

The secret is that treatment to the damaged apartment is generally best understood from the standpoint of your primary doctor, or the foreman of your apartment building. This is where all the treatment emanates, whether it be medical, surgical, or paramedical therapies (nursing). This fact of your primary doctor directing your care is so important that it will undermine all other endeavors unless your care is done through this vehicle. Why? Because this person knows you the best. Your doctor knows your medical problems, what medications you are on, your clinical status, your financial situation, your social and family issues, your personal health history, and your strengths and weaknesses.

Your doctor, because of this understanding, is, therefore, in the best position to determine the proper therapy and coordinate it all, since therapy depends on all these factors. If you lack this component, then you are going to be in deep trouble. I analogize this to an orchestra with expert, professional musicians who in and by themselves sound terrible as they warm up until the *conductor* coordinates their overall performances. Then, and only then, can a complicated musical piece sound so beautiful.

Medical treatments many times require medications. They are chemicals that we use to correct a problem in order to rectify a damaged apartment complex and return it to its normal function, or homeostasis. The secret in using a medication is that your doctor recommends it on the basis of benefit versus risk—from a simple aspirin tablet to cancer chemotherapy—because medications all have inherent risks. Some risks are small, some are large, but always remember that the decision is a weighted one, and your doctor accepts the risk of being wrong, which is called medical malpractice.

In addition, the choice of medicine should also be weighed against social, personal, and financial problems, among others. Your doctor shouldn't prescribe medication that you cannot afford. A well-kept secret that we take for granted sometimes is that the practice of medicine is a serious and dangerous business. Therefore, you want someone who will be your best advocate. Why take added risks when you are sick already? The doctor's interest in you must be measured along with his or her expertise; experience; intelligence; and, finally, availability, because if not available, he or she is worthless!

All this also holds true for surgical therapy. If you need a surgical procedure, the secret is that surgery is always a last resort and is only needed when optimal medical therapy has failed. Then your primary-care physician will decide who is the best choice to do the surgery and when. This decision will be made on the basis of who is best qualified as far as training and experience and who gives the best surgical results, along with what is best suited for your personality and financial needs.

In your apartment complex, your handyman or subcontractor has to be best suited for the job, and your own doctor is again in the best position to make this decision. Who would know better? Searching from unorthodox sources such as medical societies, ads in the newspaper, hospitals, a neighbor, the Internet, or even "brand name" institutions for surgeons is the incorrect way to go about this and can be a recipe for disaster. It only stands to reason that your physician knows the inner sanctums of the medical profession locally and can and does use the best doctors. Besides, sending you to bad doctors would only destroy his or her own practice, which would be counterproductive. Don't believe publications that include the "best" doctors in a particular area since they are nothing but self-promoting ads that are paid for by the doctor who advertised.

I have had patients misled by ads they read from various media sources and have regretted it. In my opinion, institutions with national and international reputations should be reserved for patients who have unusual or rare problems. These clinics are then referred to as true tertiary institutions, but only after a referral by your primary-care physician who has worked you up and felt that a truly higher center is necessary to solve the problem. For example, perhaps only once or twice a year, I will send a patient to a tertiary care center like the Mayo Clinic; the reason why this number is so low is that we now have in our community all university-trained physicians who have come through these same training programs and are just as qualified to take care of these complicated problems.

The only secret advantage that the tertiary institutions have are their research facilities and study protocols where medications are being used that have not been FDA approved yet, and their research teams for rare and unusual problems.

One of the problems that I have with managed care and HMOs is that they do not allow you to pick your doctor outside their network of contracted physicians, which is not a secret. As a result, they also may not allow your primary-care physician to send you to the best specialist available. In addition, they also may not allow you to go to the best institutions for whatever subspecialty care you may need unless it is in their network. So ask what the best nutrients for my condition are.

If you sense any obstruction or unreasonable restriction, go elsewhere. Like our government's state secrets, on nuclear codes your health care will depend on its *freedom*. Yes, that conductor, your doctor, will make sure that your medical care is a thing of beauty because you don't want to live in a run-down, decrepit apartment complex with substandard contractors.

The same thing holds true for surgery. We assume that when we have surgery, whatever is being done is best for us, but this may not be true. Therefore, the surgical secret is that you need to make sure that you ask relevant questions and that your primary-care doctor makes sure that you are not being fooled. I am speaking about the in-between materials and devices such as a pacemakers, prostheses, joint replacements, dentures, hearing aids, or other things that are not state-of-the-art, but cheaper. We now have a huge scandal involving cheap hip prostheses (not titanium) that wear out or don't function properly and have to be replaced. Also, dental implants that are made of cheap iron eventually start to rust.

Behind the scenes, you will find that some insurance plans will only pay for cheaper devices, and that's what you get. Your doctor and surgeon should protect you from this, but ask specifically about the device being used: Is it the best? What is it made of? How long will it last? Are there better choices or options?

As we move through the surgical-medical treatments, you can see that the whole process of diagnosing and treating becomes much more complicated than first realized. If you have several conditions at the same time; are taking eight, ten, or twelve medications; and seeing multiple specialists, then you will need a team of doctors to take care of you. It's like several apartments having multiple problems (such as with their electricity, plumbing, and air conditioning), so you must never forget that your primary-care doctor is your main go to person or general building contractor. The contractor will call in whatever team members he or she needs on the basis of quality, will conduct and coordinate their activities, and will make all major decisions with this team. Last but not least, your doctor will need the freedom to choose what is best for you!

You should also consider the possibility of death, since we all will die, and you need to consider the options you have surrounding your death before you get critically ill. The secret here includes CPR (cardiopulmonary resuscitation) or any other life-sustaining mechanism that may be used to keep you alive, which is addressed as part of a living will. My recommendation is that decisions should be made through an attorney who does most of your family's legal work, with one copy of your living will or advance directive kept in the physician's office, one with the attorney, one at home, and one in the safety-deposit box.

The secret here is to make sure you have one in hand when you go to the hospital, so there will be no question as to what to do in case of an emergency. Many times in the emergency room (ER), or during a cardiac arrest while a patient is being brought to the hospital, end-of-life decisions have to be made. If there are no legal documents available, then everything will have to be done, including mechanical ventilation. It's like carrying out a specific maintenance contract or warranty on all your apartments that has to be done *before* the need arises. Once on these life-sustaining modalities, it is very difficult to get off them. Decisions become a big problem for the family, especially if they can't agree. You might wake up in a state that was not part of your life plan, which could be a long-term disaster.

Every day, medical care and other treatments are being pushed more and more to outpatient facilities. We see outpatient surgical services, invasive diagnostic x-ray services, endoscopies, and also physical therapy with heart exercise programs all being set up on an outpatient basis. These are an integral part of your medical care and may need to be considered depending on your overall therapy. Just as important as medications or surgery, these services are all ordered by your primary-care physician and are useful adjuncts to your medical care, so make sure your insurance will pay for them.

The secret is to ask: Where are the facilities, and will your insurance pay for one near your home—not across town in a run-down facility? Also ask about how many visits are covered, because if insurance only pays for a total of three visits, it's worthless, because ordinarily you will need three times a week for six to twelve weeks to have effective therapy. If the therapy is in an unsuitable facility, you won't go. It's a shame that you need to know these in-between secrets, but with the insurance industry out of control, you had better know what to ask and what to expect.

Parenthetically, I need to mention a secret regarding side effects of medication. If you are on medication, I think that physicians need to warn you about the possible side effects if they are dangerous. But for the most part, however, I don't like telling patients about side effects because then they develop them, which is known as "medical-school diseases." It is much better to say to the patient, "Take this medication, and if you have any problems, *call me*." That is why your physician should have a phone service that will directly patch you to him or her, instead of a menu telling you to go to an ER.

Here in Florida, it is now required that the patient get a readout of the medication, and the pharmacist tells the patient of all the "evil" side effects, which scares them to death, and many times they end up not taking the medication before they get back to seeing their doctor. This can lead to very harmful, deadly effects. Another secret aspect is that doctors will often give patients medication to see what effects they may have, because this empirically will help him or her to make a diagnosis. If you don't take the medications, the doctor won't know.

Again, my position on side effects is to ask your doctor if there are any significant side effects. If the answer is no, fine. Look at it this way. Driving your car to the corner store to pick up a gallon of milk carries a risk of a fatal car accident, but we don't consider that since it is a trivial risk, and we need the milk for that particular moment. You accept the risk without really considering it. What if you were given a readout, however, that told you that you could die from an accident? Would you go to pick up the milk anyway?

In summary, as you can see, the common denominator and ultimate secret to your overall treatment, whether it be medical, surgical, or paramedical with these ancillary services, is all done through your primary-care physician—the main man or woman. If you don't have one, get one, and make sure that the doctor is not encumbered by companies or other institutions telling him or her what to do to save money. Since you cannot go to medical school to know what is right or wrong with therapies, the next best things is to have a doctor who will be your surrogate, confidant, and partner to your good health. Get the best general contractor you can for your apartment complex!

Six

The Secrets of Choosing Your Doctor (General Contractor)

There are certain things during one's life that are critical decisions. Your spouse, where you live, and your education are a few, but perhaps the most important is choosing your doctor. The reason why should be apparent because, with him or her, it could be a life-or-death decision. This may sound a bit melodramatic, but I can assure you that it is a very big decision.

In the previous chapter I mentioned insurance as being number one on your priority list in giving your doctor the freedom to choose what is best for you. The second secret is who should be your physician, which sounds simple, but it can be problematic.

From the prior chapter you now know that you need to ask yourself what's important for you and your family in regard to your overall medical care and to your good health. You obviously need a physician advocate—someone who is going to take an interest in you; who is well trained; who understands the human side of illnesses; and who is also interested in your personal problems, including finances. You want someone who practices both preventive (before you get sick) medicine but also event (when you get sick) medicine and, last but not least, is available. I remember one of my medical-school professors once saying, "No matter how smart and good a doctor is, he is worthless if not available"—not just from nine o'clock to five o'clock.

You know that your body is an integrated system of apartments, one that incorporates many, many different physiological (chemical and hemodynamic) states and one that may have several different diseases going on at the same time that also require many medications. Superimposed on this can be psychological, personal, and financial problems, with an array of tertiary considerations (religion and gender, for example), which cloud things even further. Last, you want to find a physician who is sympathetic and has empathy for your problems.

The secret is what approach you should use in looking for a doctor. First, ask other people in your neighborhood and your friends what kinds of medical problems they have had and whom they have used. Here are some of the most important questions. Ask them specifically how they feel personally about their doctor. For example, do they feel a closeness and can they count on and trust him or her? Can they reach the doctor, or does the doctor only have an automated-menu answering service telling the caller to go to the ER for emergencies or important questions, in which case he or she is not the doctor for you? Can they talk to the doctor directly, person to person, on weekends and after closing hours? Does the doctor communicate with patients and try to understand the nature of their problems, or just sit and type with their new electronic medical records? Would they invite the doctor over for dinner?

These are the questions that measure the objectiveness and subjectiveness of someone who would care for you; the answers to these questions show accountability in these areas that translates to the quality of medical care that you would receive. Basically, in summary, look for a general contractor with an established record and caring personality who is available.

Let me warn you about another secret that's not so obvious. It has been shown that male and female physicians deliver the same level of services to both genders; therefore, don't seek out a male doctor just because you are a man or seek out a female doctor just because you are a woman. Seek out a physician who will care for you and be responsive to your needs *regardless of gender*. Medical-school educations do not show preference in regard to gender or teach gender preference, which makes the gender thing a myth and only a marketing tool to get patients.

Yes, medical diseases can present differently if you are a man or women, and, yes, there are different diseases particular to gender, but in medical school, we doctors learn all of that. To me, the gender issue is just a gimmick that undermines the medical care for the entire family, and I can guarantee you that we are not trained according to gender preferences. I have seen the worst care being delivered by female doctors to female patients, and vice versa.

Education is just as important, and the secret is that the doctor has to be well trained and well rounded (that's not a reference to his or her physique). That would include not only medical school, but residency and fellowship training, together with a rich clinical experience. If the doctor has a limited, narrow training history, so their practice of medicine and expertise will also be narrow. Also, you might ask what was the doctor's undergraduate degree was in, because a strictly science person without any humanities tends to be cold and sterile. My majors were psychology and chemistry—perfect for patient care and medicine.

Going further into the depths of secrets, the doctor should be trained in an accredited institution, both for medical school and specialty training, and it would also be nice if he or she were board certified. Over the years, however, I have known many very good and well-qualified physicians who have had the necessary training but were not board certified. Therefore, this for me is a very "soft" indication for choosing a physician. I don't know why physicians do not become board certified if they are board eligible, but there may be extenuating circumstances, and, of course, this is only a measure of another examination. The most important thing is that the doctor was board eligible and has the other prevailing qualities that I have talked about.

Foreign medical-school training can also be quite misleading in choosing your doctor. More importantly, your doctor should have American specialty training in accredited institutions and speak English. However, I have seen both foreign doctors who are excellent physicians, and American graduates (of Harvard and Yale) who were terrible. Again, this is a "soft" requirement and not absolute. Use it only in the context of other things that I have reviewed for you.

There is also a great deal of confusion in regard to the titles *MD* versus *DO*. The secret is that it is partly a result of history, along with misinformation, jealousy, and prejudice. I myself am a hybrid—both a DO (osteopath) and MD (allopath) in that my medical degree is DO, but my internal medicine and GI are MD with board certification with the AMA (America Medical Association). Osteopathic training is identical to the MD, with the exception of the approach to patients and manipulation. A DO is more holistic (deals with the whole person) and tends to treat all problems, while the MD is more segmented: different doctors for different diseases.

The training programs are identical, and I know this for a fact since I've been trained in both and taught in both. The degree and board-certification exams are also identical, as are state licensure requirements. The end result for you is a choice. If are you looking for a holistic approach with perhaps manipulation, then you might prefer a DO over an MD. I've seen both excellent MD and DO physicians and terrible MD and DO physicians, so the degrees can be misleading. Therefore, you should not let the degrees persuade you, but let the other criteria that I've outlined be more important. I took no chances and got both!

I think it is also important that the physician who is taking care of you have hospital privileges. The secret here is that in order to get these privileges, a doctor needs to pass a rigorous admission process, which helps sort out many of the bad things that could have gone unnoticed. In the event that you become sick and need to be hospitalized, you obviously want this doctor to be there for psychological and medical reasons and be a vital part of orchestrating your care, especially if the problems become very complicated and dangerous to your overall well-being.

When you need your doctor the most, it's important to have the one who knows you best! There is nothing worse than going to a hospital sick and being confronted with a group of strange doctors who have no idea who you are. They don't even know what drugs you are on, what medical problems you have had in the past and worse, they don't even call your primary doctor to find out or ask about other important things regarding your medical problems.

Now, there are hospital-paid doctors that they call hospitalists. They have become very pervasive in the care that you will receive once hospitalized, but I have my reservations about them because all that I am seeing are salaried doctors not wanting to work beyond their nine-to-five because they will not receive any more money for the extra work. As a matter of fact, lawsuits in the hospitals have gone up by 30 percent as a result. As incredible as it may seem, many times we primary providers don't even know that our patients were admitted to the hospital or discharged because of the lack of communication by the hospitalists.

You also need to know another a hidden secret: that medical schools teach doctors a vast amount of didactic material, but this really does not give them the essence of community medicine and how to practice—what I call the "savvy of medicine." This takes years to develop, and some physicians never get it. The secret is that the best physician for you, in my opinion, would be one who is highly qualified, has been out in the community for at least five to ten years with the acquired "savvy," and has a commonsense experience to handle all your needs.

In my opinion, in regard to group practices, the secret is that small groups of one to three doctors are the most efficient and best for you. You don't want a large group practice where there is what I call a "rotisserie service," where you see a different doctor every day. They pass you around like a hot potato, which drives up medical costs. Also, with so many doctors who have different levels of expertise (and who don't talk to each other), the intimate care that you want will be lost. Insurance companies call that "ping-ponging," and they monitor it for unnecessary care, which is also very expensive. Five doctors taking care of you when you only need one! The end result is that you will be treated like a sheep and herded around to various corrals to see different doctors, which is not necessary and is terribly disruptive to your care and costs.

"Different doctors" are the key, and you won't see this in a small-group practice. Besides, people want to be treated like human beings, not sheep or cattle, and don't enjoy being considered just a number or part of the herd. If you have any doubt, there is also a direct relationship with continuity of care and quality of care. Who knows what is next—a bar code tattooed on the back of your head, as if you were salami at the grocery store?

Another vitally important secret for you and your family would be the number of services that the doctor offers in the office, or "under one roof," as I like to refer to it. For example, in our office, we have x-rays, heart-monitoring capabilities, blood drawing for labs, pulmonary function, PAP tests, pelvic exams, EKGs, echocardiograms, ultrasounds, Doppler, and more. It's an all-purpose office. As a result, less than 1 percent of our patients are referred elsewhere for any of these modalities, which is vitally important when you are sick and don't want to be passed off to other institutions for what needs to be done. You don't want to be sitting in the office and waiting with pain, fever, or what have you when all you want is to be home.

Our constant emphasis is total care under one roof. Also, with all this shuffling around, it is very difficult to get results to your doctor in a timely manner. In my office, I have all results within twenty-four hours, and all the services can be done within twenty minutes instead of hours spent traveling around and waiting. That includes results from CT scans and MRIs, which I have in three hours! My x-rays are read again by a radiologist, and because the result is digital, I can send images directly to the radiologist. Within three hours, I have a written report back in my office. Now that's service and can only benefit my patient care.

We also allocate sample medications and nutrients in our office to help patients defray pharmacy visits and costs. The secret for the patients is that they can avoid enormous hassles, such as waiting for two to three hours for their medications and paying exorbitant prices, many times more than the doctor visit. Even though we e-mail all our prescriptions, the pharmacies lose them, resulting in no medication when the patient gets there and more delays. The end result is that the patient becomes even more unhappy and distraught because of the stress, which can only make his or her medical conditions worse.

The secret—one worth repeating—is that all services need to be under one roof. Therefore, in summary, I would seek out a medical practice whose office offers all kinds of medical services because, if you don't, it will lead to inconveniences at the worst time (when you are sick) and be much more expensive.

You also need to make sure (a repeated secret) that your doctor is going to be available, and, yes, it is worth repeating. Find out specifically what happens at night and on the weekend, and who is covering the practice. If you find out that the doctor many times is not available, and that he or she is shipping out those types of responsibilities to other parties, I would strongly recommend that you avoid this doctor. A nine-to-five doctor will not help you at 6:00 p.m. Try this:

call the office on weekends or at night to see what happens, but don't forget, however, that a doctor needs time off too.

Also, ask specifically which emergency room to go to if trouble arises, and make sure the emergency room is near your home, not across town. The last but not least secret is to find out who will see you in the office—the doctor, physician assistant, or nurse practitioner. Do not assume it will be a doctor just because this person wears a white coat, because patients are often fooled by the people in white coats who aren't doctors (misrepresentation?). They do this a lot in urgent-care centers.

A rare secret that you've not heard before in finding a doctor is to check the waiting room, magazines, equipment, exam rooms, and even the types of patients. Is the office clean, updated, neat, and efficient? What do the other patients look like? Is there music playing? Complimentary coffee or tea? What does the office itself sound or smell like? Is it loud and hostile, or soft and friendly? What is the waiting-room conversation like, and are other patients happy or complaining?

Just sit there and listen. Observe what the staff look and act like. Do they act professionally? What do the magazines reflect, because generally they are what interests the doctor and are, therefore, a reflection of him or her? A worn-out *Field & Stream* magazine from 1990 tells you a lot. That's that old expression, "What you see and hear is what you get." I might add, is the office a happy place or a sad place? Generally speaking, that is how the office will affect you.

One last thing: for fifteen years I have used "dog power," by keeping three toy poodles in the office at all times. They wander around and add a certain energy and charm that is hard to explain, because when they are not there, you can feel the difference. Patients and their families alike (especially their kids) love them, and it puts their "psyche" at rest.

Finally, a more general secret is your physician's role in the community. All too often, physicians become so involved in their medical practices and other interests that they become totally oblivious to their surroundings and do not contribute back to the community where they live. Two hundred years ago, physicians were an integral part of any community and contributed to them heavily, not only from a medical standpoint, but socially too and, therefore, were involved in important decision-making for the community.

Ask what community activities the doctor and the doctor's family are involved in and what public service he or she has done. Personal commitment means a lot because it generally will translate the same back to you! Bottom line: I think that a responsible physician should have interplay and take an active role in the community that he or she lives in and serves medically. A good example of this is to ask if he or she lectures to various groups, what groups, and how often. Does the doctor offer other public services free and treat indigent patients or veterans, and has the doctor or the doctor's family been politically active? These are a measure of the doctor's character that translates to his or her commitment to you.

In summary, these broad, sweeping secrets will help you in choosing someone who will care for you, will be qualified to do so, and will be your advocate. If measured properly, there will never be a question of your doctor's interest, which will lead to the best care that you can possibly have.

Finally, medicine is like religion. You have to have faith and a conviction that your doctor's recommendations and level of care will guarantee you and your family the highest quality of life that can possibly be achieved. But remember, even with all of this, bad things do happen, because death is also part of living, and it's best done with someone in whom you believe and have "faith." Dying, as we all must do, with dignity will also require a physician to help you and your family through it, since dying is such a personal thing, and if you have a caring physician, even dying becomes bearable. We can all face death with a certain amount of courage and dignity.

The bottom-line secret is to choose your physician wisely, and you too will live longer, with a good quality of life, and will die, as we must, in peace with courage and dignity. Those in search of a Dr. Kevorkian have chosen unwisely and will deserve what they get.

Eight

THE SECRETS OF MEDICAL INFORMATION

*P*eople are hungry for medical information, but because of their inexperi-
ence and gullibility, they are frequently misled by parties that are just trying
to sell something. Celebrities add to the confusion because they don't have an
ounce of medical acumen, but their name recognition sells. An outline for the
nonmedical person to enrich himself or herself and not be taken to the cleaners
is this chapter's mission.

This chapter, in many ways, is rewarding for me, since it is directly related
to my live radio experience on WJNO in West Palm Beach, Florida, for twenty years and TV programming for *Fox 10 O'Clock News*. From Monday through
Friday for eight years, I did a two- to three-minute med-line, or short story, with
my toy poodle Patrick. There is obviously a great thirst for medical information,
and people are legitimately trying to find it, but the medical industry is so full of
information—some good, some bad, and some intentionally misleading—that
you might choose the wrong road to follow.

The secret in reviewing medical information is to sort out the garbage
from what is valuable information, so that you do not fall victim to a sales gimmick. The reverse is even more troublesome for me, where people who really
care get misled and tired of all the BS and say, "To heck with it!" They become

desensitized and eventually develop an "I don't care" attitude, becoming drop-outs—lost medical souls in this arena of information.

The approach that I would advise you to use is the approach that I used in reviewing for my radio and TV medical programs, which requires an understanding of what the article is really saying. The first secret step, whether you are reading the *New England Journal of Medicine* or *Vogue*, is to find out where the study originated and who the authors are. You can be fooled, however, unless you "dig" further, since Harvard studies can be erroneous too.

The second secret is to look at the study profile. The more controlled the study is, the better it is. Controlled means the treatment groups are matched equally (placebo groups and study groups with real medication) for age, sex, weight, blood pressure, and other measures. See if the study is "blind," in that the patient and investigators don't know what the patients are receiving. Finally, a crossover means that the investigators study the patients this way for a period of time and then switch the treatments/placebo groups (again blind) to see their effect. In other words, the placebo group would then get the drug, and the controlled group would get the placebo.

In contrast, retrospective studies are studies that go back and review data to draw conclusions, but they are unreliable since they lack controls. Finally, a meta-analysis is a retrospective study of several older studies with conclusions derived. This too lacks control, but the older studies' sheer volume and similarities are better than the single retrospective one.

I would be remiss if I didn't mention anecdotal data where an individual case is reported. For example, "Mr. Jones took this and got better." These are worthless in and by themselves (testimonials), since they do not control important variables, which can lead to erroneous conclusions and most times show a deliberate bias. You see these testimonials all the time in ads and on TV and the Internet, but ironically, many times, these reports—if legitimate—will then lead to a better-controlled study because of the interest, and then, and only then, reliable data and conclusions may be derived.

Another hidden secret is to take a look at who sponsored the study. For example, I recently reviewed two articles having to do with salt and high blood pressure. One from the United Kingdom reported that a low-salt diet would benefit and not hurt you if you had high blood pressure, and one in the United States said just the opposite. How would you solve the dilemma with contradictory results? Looking carefully at the small print, however, revealed that the US study was sponsored by the Campbell's Soup company (problem solved: soups have high sodium contents), and the other study had no commercial relationships. Watch for the conflicts of interest.

In addition, you have to be especially careful about reading articles in the newspaper. The secret with newspapers is that they are engineered for one purpose and one purpose only—to *sell newspapers.* They assume no responsibility for content, deliberately try to embellish certain features of an article to catch your attention, and almost always editorialize their own political or social beliefs in the article. I have found the newspaper, along with the Internet, to be particularly dangerous for all these reasons. Don't be used by these sources, because the profiteers will laugh all the way to the bank, but this is not to discourage you. I think you need to read, as I do, with a broad range of subjects, but without the naïveté that will lead you in the wrong direction.

Finally, when you read medical articles, especially in newspapers, read the whole article beyond the headline, and be suspicious of anything that makes no sense. If you have any questions, ask your doctor and bring the article in for him or her to review.

Over the years, people will say to me, "Your radio/TV programming is advertising, isn't it?" My response was that I didn't use the programs as a way of patronizing my medical practice, and I clearly tried to keep it as a public service. But indirectly, when people hear you and assess your medical ability and personality, over time, they will come to you if they are unhappy with their own present medical situation. There can be many reasons why someone would want to leave a doctor, which can include a poor office staff (someone was rude); noncaring office personnel can be a game changer. I really don't believe that doctors need to advertise, but you will see ads all the time. Generally, these are big groups or companies that can afford it. My position has always been to let your reputation precede you, and it hasn't changed, which works very well.

What I am saying is that advertising can be done by a physician or physicians' groups in a way that is constructive and as a public service. At the same time, this has benefits for them because they can get the feedback necessary to assess their own job efficiency. I can honestly say that after twenty years on the radio, eight years on Fox TV, and thirty-seven years of medical practice, I have learned a lot about people, their illnesses, and their interrelationships. Taking care of patients, in my office and at the hospital; curing them; and also seeing them die is the majority of what I do, but I think in the end that public communication means even more to me because I can touch so many other people.

In summary, these secrets may seem simplistic, but you will find that they should be the quintessential framework for your overall care. I think that sometimes we are all overwhelmed and inundated with information. As a result, we cannot see the forest for the trees. A recent trip to Barnes and Noble only confirmed for me the dilemma for the average consumers who want to take care of themselves and their families by learning as much as possible and becoming informed consumers. It really is sad! So many books saying so many different things, along with the Internet and TV—it even confuses someone in the business like yours truly.

Eight

THE SECRETS OF MEDICATION

When a doctor prescribes a medication for you, the doctor has assumed the responsibility for it, along with weighing the benefits versus the risks. You also assume responsibility for taking it as prescribed and also for the handling of it properly, which requires a fundamental knowledge of chemistry. Medicine in all aspects is a two-way street, and medication is a perfect example.

The first secret is that the one thing that we take for granted is our medication. We carelessly store it in the wrong place. Many times we don't even take it or don't take it as prescribed (say, two instead of three times a day), and then when we do take it, we take it with everything other than water, even with alcohol! Don't forget that the medication that we are supposed to take is largely responsible for why our life expectancies have almost doubled in the last fifty years. We should worship the very ground that drug researchers stand on, along with the drug companies that researched and developed them. For example, look at serious infections like MRSA (methicillin-resistant staphylococcus aureus) and the antibiotics to treat it. The same is true for the newer heart medications.

Did you know that one drug costs about half a billion to one billion dollars to research and develop, but only one drug out of nine makes it to the marketplace? With the politicians and the media bad-mouthing the drug companies, it's a wonder that they are still in this country, although many have left for overseas sites, which has cost us millions of jobs and tax dollars.

If you have an advancing cancer, you will know what I'm talking about, because when your doctors run out of drugs that are available or in the pipeline, you will die, and that's it. We need to keep this pipeline of drugs coming, and it will only do that with a capitalist system (research and development) that rewards innovation. Most drug companies take 10 percent of their gross revenues and use it for this very thing. That's a lot of money that could be profits.

Over the years I have seen a "plague effect," where the entire medical system is shutting down because of our politicians and the White House placing unwarranted restrictions and laws in the way of innovation and the practice of medicine in general. Our medical care is still the finest in the world, but it may not be for long, and that includes our drug-manufacturing companies too. We cannot allow the government to kill it so that they can take it over. Oh my God, the VA hospital care for all of us!

Those of us over a certain age can all remember the pharmacist mixing and preparing prescriptions with his mortar and pestle, but now we have an automated pill-delivery system with technicians, and the pharmacist is not even in the pharmacy. Yes, scattered around are compounding pharmacies that principally do bioidentical hormones the old-fashioned way, but unfortunately, these are a gimmick. You don't need someone grinding away to get identical hormones (that are not really identical), which already come in a pill and are regulated and controlled the FDA.

The secret is that, in that little pill or capsule that the doctor prescribes, there is a huge amount of research that was done to make sure that you receive a measured dose of the active ingredient, which is then bioavailable to the tissues that are its target organs. This all has to be predictable, with a reliable response; otherwise, the drug will not be approved.

How the preparation in a pill, capsule, or liquid is added to other ingredients or adjuvants is very important and has become a serious problem with generic medications that poorly control these variables. The only thing that they need is the active ingredient, available to the target cells in adequate amounts. But it turns out that the active ingredient, even in adequate amounts, will not work as it should if the adjuvants or add-ons don't allow it to, and that's the big difference between generic and trade drugs.

It's surprising that the technology is so little understood and appreciated, because even how the active ingredient is placed in or on the tablet (on the surface and leached off), time released, or encapsulated behind several layers requires a great deal of research, extremely bright people, and dollars to do it. I have had patients tell me that the pill was found in their stool, but what they didn't realize is that the active ingredient was on the surface and digested off, and only the wax carrier was left because it is indigestible.

When it comes to drugs and insurance plans, you now enter the secret world of profit. Insurance plans that cover medication do not look at its effectiveness or what's best for you. They look at money saved! As I like to say, you can kiss that off, and the same is true for laboratory coverage. The insurance companies use the labs that cut them the best deal and again kiss off your interest, so let me give you example.

We have a local lab here that returns results to me and calls if there is a critical test, by the next morning for the lab tests drawn the prior day. Because the lab didn't cut a deal with some of the other insurance plans, its patients are forced to go to a draw station somewhere else, with limited hours, and then I don't get the results for three to four days. To make it worse, most times results are not complete because the insurance-based lab has lost the requisition or because their help does not speak English, and they have made a mistake. That is lousy service, injurious to the patient, and all for profit. The secret is: who cares that the lab ties up my nursing staff forever to get the results being passed from one person to another, who are probably sitting right next to each other! Even when physicians try to expedite their care to help patients, the profiteers (insurance companies) then threaten us with disenrollment and tell us what to do.

When you are given a medication, the doctor has the responsibility for prescribing it correctly, from the dose to its clinical indications, and you have the responsibility for taking it correctly. A very subtle secret is that the doctor needs to also consider your pocketbook and the drug's efficacy (how effective is it) and then match them so as not to waste your time and theirs. An expensive, effective drug that is unaffordable is useless.

Here are some secret guidelines: First, all new drugs are expensive. I don't care how many coupons they offer you, or how detailed the song and dance about its virtues is, it will be expensive. It takes time for the insurance companies to catch up—years—so even though it's the greatest drug since sliced bread, it is expensive. Number two, don't let the VA hospital be your guide. The reason is that the federal government, in order to save money, uses the cheapest medications and uses medications that I haven't used for twenty years. Older drugs, of course, are not as good as the more recent medications with more side effects, but the VA doesn't care. It's only our vets! You can add this to denying care and then falsifying records.

On the other hand, in dealing with patients who have the money, it sometimes becomes a bit confusing because costs can be very relative. Let me give you an example. You would think that wealthy patients who are educated and can afford it would want the best of care, including the best of medications. Well, think again! I recently had a patient who sold his company for $100 million and was taking a three-month golfing trip by private jet around the world, but who refused to pay for a medication because it was too expensive! So you can see, no matter how much money you have, it's a matter of priorities.

When I decide on what is affecting my patients, I generally give them a choice and explain the differences. After all, it's their choice, so they need all the facts to make an informed decision. Now, magnify that by the other drugs that they may be taking, and you can see that some massaging or adjustment may be necessary to get all the drugs aboard.

One little trick when the drugs are the same price, no matter the dose, is to order the higher dose and tell patients to cut the pill in half. That will decrease the cost of that drug by 50 percent. If it's a capsule, tell the patient to empty half the contents into applesauce and then eat it. (Some long-acting drugs [LA on the label], however, cannot be cut in half because their blood levels are predicated on the whole dose being delivered at once. That means that if the bottle says "long-acting," you can't split it; if you have any questions, ask your doctor.) The applesauce will cut any unfavorable taste but will not affect the drug itself. This little trick works also for patients who cannot swallow pills or capsules. If there is a liquid alternative, then ask for it, but many drugs do not come in a liquid form.

Let me finish this train of thought with this. Don't believe for one minute that your insurance company, in its approved drug list, has chosen these drugs because they are the best ones. Some drugs are, but some are not, and you will find out that many times the insurance companies will choose drugs on the basis on how much money the drug company kicked back to the insurance company. This is especially prevalent with mail orders and three-month suppliers. The kickback amount is key here (could be hundreds of thousands of dollars) and not what drug is best for you. When I see this disparity, I tell the patient that this approved drug is not the best one, why, and then let him or her choose. I, of course, verify all of this in my office note so that later on, the patient cannot not claim that I didn't prescribe what was best for him or her. Remember this: it's the doctor's responsibility to advise the patient which drug is best for the patient, not based on the cost. It's the patient's responsibility to choose and then pay for the drug.

There is a secret psychology in taking medications, and it goes something like this: the more you take, the worse off you are. I have seen this to be especially true with my diabetics who are reluctant to take insulin because if they think that if they are taking it, they're worse off. The same often occurs with cardiac patients taking their medications. With these patients, where sudden death is a consideration, this could be a fatal judgment. With diabetics, their complication rates are directly related to their blood sugar control, so no matter how many drugs are being used, control is king, which we measure with the blood A1C level that measure blood sugars over thirty to ninety days. My recommendation would be that when your doctor requests that you take more medication, ask why, but don't automatically say no. Psychology plays a large role in taking medications, but for drugs to be effective, our goal is to overcome that fear.

Another big psychological secret factor is the placebo effect. I will touch on this later, but I see no problem in using it with my patients to get a desired effect. If I can instill in the patient a feeling that what we are doing will help him or her, then my chances of success will only be that much greater. Look at the reverse, the "nocebo" effect. If I tell that same patient that what we are doing probably will not work, how much success will we have? Confidence and hope in winning not only applies in sports, but in health care too, and I have found that when patients lose hope, everything is lost. Even drugs and nutrients that I know should be helping won't help; that old expression about mind over matter is so true.

A more recent problem with medications is with preauthorization. I will write a prescription for a patient, and the insurance company will refuse to pay for it unless we fill out forms to justify it. Do you know how much time my staff spends writing out forms and with phone calls as a result of this? The secret is that this paperwork is nothing more than a form of rationing, and it puts the doctor between the patient and the insurance company. We suddenly are now the employees of the insurance company and are responsible for getting the prescription, which they pay us zero for, and yet we are spending many dollars every day for our staff to chase these drug preauthorization's down.

The other secret of this is, of course, the patients' feeling that it is the doctor's responsibility to "get 'er done," like Larry the Cable Guy says. We do our best, and delays do occurs purely because the insurance companies cut deals with drug companies.

There is another secret reality that sometimes you need to pay for your medications, like that car, cruise, casino, TV, and so on. As the screw tightens with the Affordable Care Act, and as the rationing becomes more obvious, you all will be involved. That metaphor regarding drug reimbursements at the end of the year, "donut hole," means that patients are not saving enough money to cover their medications. That would mean that a drug coverage by insurance would eventually run before the end of the year and you as the patient would have to pay for it.

One of the greatest secrets that I have discovered about patients and their medications is that patients don't take them. It sounds ridiculous, but even worse, they will take their medications sometimes. In this case, the medical condition is partially treated, which makes it impossible for their doctors to make any clinical decisions. Forget about that empirical test! Thank God I'm good with arithmetic, since that's how I generally catch them. When I add up their monthly allotments and see twenty pills left over, I know that patients are not taking drugs as instructed.

My father was famous for not taking his medications, but his reason was that he was cheap, and he was saving them up! I guess it went back to the Depression days that he lived through on a farm. Regardless, you need to take your medication as instructed; otherwise, you will disrupt the entire thought process in deciphering your medical problem. This is one of those situations where saving doesn't add up!

A very recent problem—one that as an American is hard for me to believe—is that we are running out of medications, especially chemotherapeutics for cancer treatment. On a trip to the Eastern bloc countries, I attended a lecture by a person who lived through both the Nazi and Russian occupations in the Czech Republic. I asked him, "What was the biggest difference between them and a democracy?" He said that the difference was that in a capitalistic system, supply and demand directed one's economy, while under the other regimens, especially the Soviets, it was demand and supply. In other words, under the Russian economy, when you saw a line of people, you would get into it because you knew that you needed whatever it was.

With rationing in this country, which goes by many other names like *authorizations*, these lines will become even more apparent, whether it be cancer medications or food. That's what a government take-over really means, demand and supply like the old Czech Republic. My prediction is that medical care will only get worse, and the lines longer, unless of course you have the cash to buy goods and services directly. There is always a market for staying well and not dying, whether it is on the black market or through the demand-and-supply method.

As we go through this transition, try to remember what it was like when there was no price discrimination. It's not unusual for patients today to go to the pharmacy and be told that their medication will be coming in next week, so make sure that you have a least two weeks' worth of medication on hand, just in case you find yourself in that line of demand and supply.

I am sure that once this book is finally printed and distributed, we will be further down the road of a government-controlled medical system, and as dreadful as it seems, it will be worse—worse because Americans are not Canadians or Europeans who are much more receptive to government intervention and control than we are—but I am also confident that there will be a large percentage of

Americans who still value their health care over their pleasure-seeking desires. There will be choices, and you will need to make them.

For example, in Germany almost 70 percent of people have additional health care coverage that they pay for out of pocket because they are not happy with the government system, which is free. Yes, they pay for the government health care through their high tax system, but the additional cost for their insurance is worth it, which they know and value. In poorer countries like Greece and Spain, the percentage is much smaller, but there still are people who want their health care when they need it and not months down the road. It's their choice, not their governments.

The British system, which is probably the oldest in one recent quality study, found dreadful woes that permeate and require total restructuring that will be impossible. The government never does health care better, and anyone who believes that is either stupid or from another planet! This niche for the private sector of medicine will in time evolve into its own prominence because the stark difference between it and the government system will be so vast that even a blind man could see the difference. It will be admired again for what it is—a field of study that delivers daily, life-sustaining, and quality-of-life instructions not found anywhere else. People ask me what I do, and I tell them, "Stamp out disease and save lives." Who else can say that?

Nine

MORE UNTOLD BASIC SECRETS—THE INTANGIBLES

There is much to medicine and its practice that falls between the lines. Crossing social, gender, mental, and economic boundaries, medical care raises other issues that need to be discussed. Because of their inherent nature—just like religion, hypnosis, and prior lives as other humans—however, these boundaries aren't even considered and are taken for granted, but can have dramatic effects on overall care.

Many things seem tangential to medicine, but in my opinion they shouldn't be. With human illness, there is so much at stake, and I feel that we should use everything in our power to help patients with and through their illnesses.

When I was doing live radio a number of years ago, I tried to bring to my audience interesting concepts or people, and many of them even fascinated me. One was Dr. Brian Weiss, who is a Yale-trained psychiatrist in Miami. That in of itself is not too exciting, but what he did was. In his book, *Many Lives, Many Masters*, he describes patients who under hypnosis went on to describe in great detail prior lives. They spoke foreign languages under hypnosis that they had no present-day knowledge of, and one spoke a dead language that hadn't been spoken for five hundred years. It surprised Weiss greatly. With disbelief when it kept happening patient after patient, he kept a log and then wrote books about his patient's experiences.

Some of the questions that I asked him included these: Can you come back in the opposite sex? (His answer: No.) What was the most famous person in a prior life? (His answer: A Napoleon general.) Are you in prior lives with family members and favorite animals? (His answer: Yes, but in much different contexts.)

It's this secret landscape of the semi mystical that I want to wrap this book around, if possible, along with the hard, standardized medical facts.

In medicine there are many things that are secrets, and we cannot explain them all. Any doctor who says otherwise needs further self-examination, or he or she has been to Walt Disney World one too many times. If you advise a patient to do certain things and he or she gets better, it's because of the medication, the placebo effect, God, or all three. If you tell him or her the reverse, most times he or she will not get better, and that's called the nocebo effect.

If mind over matter, hypnosis or the power of suggestion, religion (you believe in something), mumbo jumbo, voodoo, or whatever else for me is an ally in getting patients better, then I will use it. The purest will say, of course, that this practice is misleading patients or deceiving them, but I say, "So what." As long as I'm not deceiving them for my personal benefit, and they are getting better, then it's fair game.

In my opinion, physicians use these intangibles modalities and opportunities too little, and it only hurts the patients that they are treating. For example, in my personal experience, I have found that patients who have religion to be easier to take care of because they are more compliant and more family supported. When dealing with bad medical problems, they accept them more graciously, because I guess that the human spirit needs some backup.

For those of you who think that religion is for the weak, then you are missing out, because, on the contrary, it makes you stronger. When you look at history and see the strength, courage, and bravery in the name of religion, you can see why I say that. Finally, this really comes in handy when you and your family are facing a dreadful and deadly medical problem.

As a corollary to this, I would recommend that you read *Proof of Heaven*, by Dr. Eben Alexander. A Harvard-trained neurosurgeon and professor, he contracted a severe form of meningitis, and while he was in a coma with little hope of surviving, he documented an almost-existential mind experience of going to heaven. He then explains it based on his knowledge of brain anatomy and his experience as a brain surgeon. Ask yourself, if anyone could know if this were real or not, wouldn't he be the one? He has written a sequel, but the first book's concepts fit nicely into the "intangibles" of medicine and give us perhaps more insight into the afterlife, as Dr. Weiss did.

Hypnosis goes way back in history, and the Egyptians were the first in documenting its usage, but it wasn't until the seventeenth century that Dr. Franz Mezmer, an Austrian physician, popularized it again. Sound familiar? *Mesmerization* or to be mesmerized! As you will see, hypnosis has many secrets, so let's explore them.

In regard to hypnosis, more recently, Dr. Carol Ginandes, a Harvard psychologist, asked, "If someone told you that you could treat 100 different conditions without a prescription and was free without significant side effects, would you do it?"

When hypnotized, against popular belief, you are not unconscious and not asleep, and you are open to suggestion. It's estimated that 70–90 percent of people can get into this altered state of suspended skepticism, which it is now referred to as. It's like daydreaming and focusing on a single thought with purpose, or listening to the radio in your car so intently that you don't remember diving home or how you did it.

Studies have shown that hypnosis can block pain sensations from getting to the brain, which normally interprets them through "conscious perception." PET scans show, however, that someone under hypnosis processes sounds and images the same as real ones; therefore, the brain accepts hallucinations as real. That does not happen without hypnosis. Once hypnotized, however, your brain can be fooled. For example, a bottle of perfume can be made to smell like ammonia or even worse! With this same methodology, burns could be perceived as not painful and chemotherapy as not causing nausea. In other words, let fantasy preempt these symptoms.

It's been also reported that hypnosis can expedite healing. In a group of women with reconstructive breast surgery, one group received standard therapy. The second group received standard therapy along with a therapist, and the third group received standard therapy with hypnosis. The third group healed quicker and with less pain and less pain medication.

Hypnosis was also studied at the NIH (National Institute of Health) with bone fractures, and the researchers found the same for patients who achieved greater mobility and used less medication. A Manchester, England, study of irritable bowel syndrome (IBS) reported that 80 percent of patients improved in three months using hypnosis and remained well for eight years. Their anxiety and depression decreased by 50 percent—again, requiring less medication. In addition, these studies were reproduced with IBS patients at the University of North Carolina by Dr. Olafur Palsson.

Skin conditions may also benefit, like warts of all kinds. Tulane University reported an 80 percent cure rate along with clearing of eczema, including sleep disorders, itching, and stress. One of the most obvious secrets, and perhaps one the greatest benefits of hypnosis, is in controlling pain.

At the University of Washington's burn unit, medical professionals concluded that hypnosis was beneficial for virtually every pain problem they had with their burn patients. It seems to convert the sensation of intolerable pain into another gentler, softer sensation, but does not totally replace it. In pregnant women, a study from Australia reported that hypnotized women had shortened labor and reduced pain and pain-medication use, decreased complication rates, and a shortened time of recovery. It doesn't stop here. Children who were born of hypnotized women had higher Apgar scores; therefore, they were breathing better, and mothers were less likely to have postpartum depression.

Here's a good one for me: the dentist. Many people do not go to the dentist because of the fear factor—like me. I'm no exception, but I go anyway. To deal with fear, I need the "gas" from the waiting room right into the exam room ("den of torture," I call it), right up until I leave, including paying for the visit. That makes even the paying less painful! Don't think for one minute that hypnosis will erase the need for Novocain, unless you are Hercules, but you will tolerate the procedure a whole lot easier.

In cancer patients, hypnosis will not only reduce the pain but may actually increase the life span. In a study done with breast-cancer patients, self-hypnosis decreased pain by 50 percent and increased life spans by a year and a half.

Finally, hypnosis for smoking and losing weight has been rather disappointing. I did have one patient who was a chain smoker with extreme anxiety and who did quit with the use of hypnosis, which greatly surprised me, and I told her so. But unfortunately, two years later she died of lung cancer.

After I reviewed this whole topic of hypnosis, I came to the same conclusion that you did: why isn't it being used more often? The secret, I'm certain, is that these services are not being covered by Medicare and the insurance companies, plus the doctors are not aware of the benefits. Just like insurance companies telling doctors where to send patients for their labs, the labs have cut a deal with the insurance companies, even though it's not in the best interest of the patient.

Hypnosis, in my opinion, should be a major player in your health care, but in its proper context, because it has great validity. Ask for it, and make sure you go to a person with the proper training and experience to guarantee some benefit. Your doctor would be a good place to begin for this advice, and if he or she does not know, let your provider research it for you. Even if you have to pay for hypnosis out of your own pocket, I think that it is worth it. By the way, get used to this paying for it, because with these new Obama policies and $12,000 deductibles, you will be paying up front for all your medical care, not just hypnosis.

Ten

The Secrets of Heart Disease

*H*eart disease kills more than one million Americans a year. It is the number-one cause of death. Heart disease, for all practical purposes, can be broken down into three groups: coronary heart disease, congestive heart failure, and arrhythmias (abnormal heart rhythm). So let's look at each cause, analyze it, and find nutrient therapies.

The cardiovascular system (heart and blood vessels) includes the heart (the pump) and blood vessels (arteries and veins), which are the highways that provide blood (oxygen and nutrients) to all organ systems of the body. It's basically a transportation system, and if it is interrupted because of a faulty pump or highway system, then all other organ systems will suffer. The heart, in addition, needs its own blood supply, which it gets through the coronary arteries that branch off the aorta just outside the heart.

Plaque can build up inside these arteries. The condition is called atherosclerosis, in which blood flow is interrupted. If the coronary arteries do not supply the heart adequately, a heart attack (death of heart cells) may occur. But a problem in the peripheral arteries can cause kidney failure or gangrene of the extremities. The arteries can also become enlarged, like a bubble on a tire. The enlargements are called aneurysms, which can rupture and cause sudden death. The abdominal aorta is a major concern for aneurysms, especially as we get older and when associated with hypertension (elevated blood pressure), diabetes, or elevated lipids. As the cells in the rest of the body, including the heart and blood-vessel cells, try to reproduce and replace themselves to stay healthy, these same risk factors diminish that vital function, which leads to aging, and that's why these risk factors need to be monitored with that yearly physical exam and normalized.

We are getting skilled at bioengineering our patients. Make sure that you get checked and, like the Marines, find your enemy (risk factors) and kill them (get rid of risk factors) so you're not killed first. Our son was a Marine captain, so I know, but if you wait for symptoms to occur, it's too late, and the die will have been cast.

Coronary Artery Disease

The most common cause of death from heart disease is coronary artery disease (CAD), which results from clogging of coronary arteries that deliver nutrients and oxygen to the heart tissues. Symptoms generally include chest pain, but there are many derivations of this, including having no chest pain (especially for women).

The typical chest pain that occurs with activity tends to be over the left anterior aspect of the chest. A patient may feel a heavy and squeezing sensation, associated with shortness of breathing and sweating. The pain lasts just a few minutes to begin with and then goes away, which fools the patient into thinking that the problem is not serious. There is a variant called Prinzmetal angina in which the pain occurs with rest and sleeping, not activity (the reverse), but it still is caused by the same underlying blockage problem.

Incidentally, if you or someone you are with is having a heart attack, chewing four aspirin tablets could be lifesaving. Risk factors have to be found and treated to prevent a heart attack. Just recently, a new secret was reported. Data suggest that even during an acute myocardial infarction (heart attack), carnitine, lipoic acid, taurine, and branched-chain amino acids will help limit the damage by protecting the mitochondria, which are the energy makers. That is a very recent secret, right off the press!

The secret is to prevent heart disease by finding risk factors, correcting them, and treating other medical diseases such as diabetes and hypertension that accelerated it. Your physician needs to test you for these conditions and treat them; otherwise, coronary artery disease can and will result. You can see how interrelated these conditions become.

Yearly laboratory tests would include testing for the aforementioned conditions along with advanced lipid profiles that include cholesterol, LDL, HDL, triglycerides, and non-HDL but also LPA (the widow-maker) and lipid molecular particle profiles. Also, genetic testing for heart disease is available along with CRP, an LpPLA indicator of blood-vessel inflammation, and omega-3 blood levels, which, if low, will increase the risk of heart disease.

More recently, A1C, insulin, and free fatty acids have been added as early markers of diabetes, and BNP and galectin as markers for early myocardial (heart) disease. Lastly, sterols, or plant fats, have been added to the lab testing. If elevated, these conditions need to be treated with drugs such as Zetia or Welchol, or naturally with guggal, a tree-gum extract.

These blood levels all have to be normal, and believe it or not, we can normalize them and take away any risk (through bioengineering). There have been over thirty studies to date illustrating this point, and the good news is that nutrients can be used to normalize lipids alone or in conjunction with standard medication. Just to give you an example, these secret nutrient therapies would include omega-3 oil; olive oil; red-yeast rice; lipotain (guggal extract); or policosanol, a sugar-cane extract for an elevated lipid level. Also, garlic, tocotriens, K2, and pomegranate decrease plaque buildup and actually remove what's there.

These nutrients all work by decreasing the cholesterol and LDL (the bad cholesterol) while increasing the HDL (good cholesterol), which removes plaque. In addition, the omega-3 oils, garlic, and tocotriens decrease triglyceride levels, which also remove plaque. Finally, pomegranate works through the PONS receptor (paraoxonase) on the HDL molecule, which removes plaque. It sounds very technical, and it is, but there is no reason why this bioengineering can't be part of your life.

If diabetes (which will be discussed in detail in the next chapter) is part of the scenario, then control of weight and blood sugar is mandatory, along with nutrient therapy that would include green-coffee extract, carnosine, AMPK (adenosine monophosphate kinase), and bilberry. With hypertension, Hawthorne, CoQ10, taurine, and passion flower may be used. Last but not least is obesity, which underlies all these problems. Solutions would include weight loss and an exercise program for three hours a week. Irvingia, an African mango extract, will help with the weight loss as a glucose inhibitor, which is another nutrient secret here.

You can see how complicated heart disease becomes, but if you use the next secret, a problem-oriented approach that most physicians use, the treatment will make sense and keep it organized. With the problem-oriented approach, you list the most serious condition first. Under it, you list drug treatment protocols. This system keeps track and prioritizes not only the diseases, but the medications along with treatment plans, and also helps organize your thoughts.

As we get older, the problems seem to pile up along with their treatments, and that's why they say that getting older is not for sissies. George Bernard Shaw said it best: "Youth is wasted on the young." The important secret here is that your health journey is a joint venture with your doctor, and your records are your health bible.

Congestive Heart Failure

Congestive heart failure occurs when the heart muscle becomes weak. As a result, blood has trouble flowing from left to right. Normally, blood is pumped out of the heart from the left ventricle through the aortic system via arteries to oxygenate the rest of the body. It returns back to the heart through the venous system on the right side to be oxygenated again in the lungs, and then the cycle repeats itself. That's why it is referred as left to right.

In reality, the blood is going from the left side to the right side of your body, which needs to be maintained in good health. If your heart becomes weak, it cannot keep up, and the blood reverses and goes backward—or, to say it differently, goes less forward. Blood then congests into the lungs and causes shortness of breath (dyspnea), paroxysmal nocturnal dyspnea (the patient wakes up short of breath), and orthopnea (the patient cannot lie flat and must be propped up with pillows to breathe), along with the eventual congestion in the legs with swelling (edema), which is the picture of congestive heart failure.

If not corrected, congestive heart failure can lead to pulmonary edema (water in the lungs) and death by literally drowning. There are many etiologies (causes), such as coronary artery disease, hypertension, and genetic (cardiomyopathy) heart failure, so these conditions have to be diagnosed and treated appropriately. Digitalis, beta-blocker drugs like Coreg, and diuretics like Lasix and Aldactone are our first-line treatments. They can be very effective. Recent revelations, however, having to do with muscle physiology and its energy sources have now put nutrient therapies on the front burner.

The nutrient treatment secrets are that CoQ10, PQQ, acetylcarnitine, carnitine, branched-chain amino acids, taurine, Hawthorne, and lipoic acid will maintain cardiac enzymes along with mitochondria function and will make cellular energy more productive in the heart. Recent studies now indicate that these agents help grow new mitochondria (biogenesis) in the heart, which will improve cardiac function and normalize the left-to-right blood flow.

I think that this is a good point to interrupt myself in our discussion in order to reveal a truly monumental secret. Mitochondria in every cell in our body make energy for our cells, like the gasoline tanks in our cars. This cellular energy allows our cells to function normally (heart muscle cells pump the blood) and reproduce themselves when they wear out. Every cell in our body has about two to twenty-five hundred mitochondria, and the mitochondria all have their own separate DNA and are not dependent on the cell-nucleus DNA. To make cellular energy is the key to understand heart disease and many other diseases including aging, since as we age, the number of mitochondria decease, which decreases our energy source—our gasoline for life. If we lose mitochondria, we age, and in the heart, aging leads to congestive heart failure.

Standard medications will only put a Band-Aid on the problem, whereas the nutrients preserve and actually increase in number the gasoline, or mitochondria, in our cells to improve their function. That's irony for you—nutrients work better than medications! As mentioned, medications such as Coreg (a beta-blocker), diuretics along with Aldactone, and digitalis are similarly prescribed for the heart failure (the Band-Aids).

Also, it may be a bit too technical, but I'm going to mention diastolic dysfunction. During the diastolic phase of heart function (when the chambers fill with blood), if the filling phase is incomplete, it's called diastolic dysfunction, which results in the systolic, or pumping, phase becoming dysfunctional or abnormally low. The Mayo Clinic and others have looked at diastolic dysfunction, but to date no drug class has helped. But nutrients can help. CoQ10, PQQ, carnitine, branched-chain amino acids, lipoic acid, and taurine all in unison strengthen the heart muscle to pump more effectively even during diastole, therefore normalizing systole, or blood flow, out of the heart.

Arrhythmia

The third part of heart disease is arrhythmias, or abnormal rhythms. They can cause symptoms of palpitations, vertigo (dizziness), chest pain, syncope (fainting), and shortness of breath, but they may have no symptoms and be found only on a routine physical exam. By location, arrhythmias can be atrial, nodal, or ventricular—with the atrial ones being far more common. They all can be fatal, but the nodal and ventricular ones are the most dangerous.

Drugs and pacemakers are the most frequent treatments, but with atrial arrhythmias, drugs and nutritional therapies may be very helpful. Prematurities such as premature atrial contractions (PACs) are the most common and most harmless. The next would be premature ventricular contractions (PVCs), which are also most times benign, but they can be dangerous especially if they are frequent, coupled (together), or multifocal (coming from different sources). They sometimes can progress to fatal ventricular arrhythmias such as ventricular tachycardia or ventricular fibrillation and, therefore, need immediate medical treatment.

From the atria, atrial fibrillation is next most common, and a fibrillating heart loses about 30 percent of its cardiac output. Most people can tolerate the loss and function normally—and therefore have no symptoms. They don't even know they have atrial fibrillation, which is dangerous because there is a 50 percent incidence of emboli phenomena (blood clots) to the brain, which can result in strokes over a two-year study.

Fibrillation may be treated with electrical conversion, ablation, or medications such as beta-blockers, digitalis, and amiodarone, but the nutritional secret is that the omega-3 oils are also very helpful in increasing conversion rates by 50 percent. CoQ10, PQQ, and lipoic acid may also be tried, along with taurine, which decreases sympathetic input (overstimulation). But regardless, anticoagulants like Coumadin are necessary to avoid systemic emboli (clots to the rest of the body) or strokes that can occur.

Anticoagulants are necessary because data tell us that with chronic or paroxysmal fibrillation, within two years of beginning treatment, embolic rates are decreased from 50 percent to 5 percent with anticoagulants as compared to a nontreated control group. So it's your choice. Additionally, with atrial fibrillation, any underlying condition must also be ruled out or treated, such as high blood pressure, coronary artery disease, or an overactive thyroid. I had a patient with chronic atrial fibrillation who converted spontaneously with testosterone replacement for low-T syndrome, so make sure that condition is ruled out. Now that's a twofer secret!

In summary, I now have reviewed the three most common types of heart diseases and their nutritional secret therapies. By taking these medications, including my secret nutrient ones, we must always add exercise and weight loss, if you are overweight. The exercise especially must be under your physician's guidance, since unbridled exercise with any of these problems could be fatal.

Finally, in my experience, I have seen remarkable recoveries in patients with severe heart disease from all three types because of the nutrient add-ons. They have made a great difference. For example, I had one patient with an enlarged heart (*cor bovinum*, or heart of the cow) from hypertension who couldn't even brush his teeth without getting short of breath because of congestive heart failure. With these treatment plans that I have just outlined, within one month, all his symptoms resolved, and his heart size returned to normal. The cardiologist was amazed because he had not seen anything like it.

In summary, the secret with most cardiac conditions is that you must make a diagnosis first, treat with the standard medications, and then use the nutrient add-ons with mitochondria energy as the basis. You, and the doctors too, need to think in terms of mechanisms and basic physiology, which is the way we were taught, but for some reason this emphasis was lost along the way when we, the doctors, were learning clinical medicine. From cancer to diabetes and heart disease, the basic mechanisms of nutrients make them understandable and provide a rationale for how to apply them.

Eleven

THE SECRETS OF DIABETES

In the course of my office practice every day, I probably see more patients with diabetes than those with any other disease. Therefore, just in sheer numbers, we all need to understand it and the secrets of nutritional therapies, because these therapies are major players. Ironically, almost all my colleagues in the medical profession are oblivious to nutrients, and perhaps they too will read this book.

Diabetes Mellitus

The main secret in understanding diabetes is that there are two types of diabetes. Diabetes insipidus is a brain disorder that causes an increased thirst but has nothing to do with blood sugar and the diabetes that you are aware of (diabetes mellitus). It has to do with a deficiency of an antidiuretic hormone (vasopressin) that is made by the posterior pituitary, and this condition is rare.

Diabetes mellitus, on the other hand, is a different critter, which is more dangerous, costly, and much more common. Type 1, or juvenile type, generally occurs before the age of twenty and is insulin dependent. People with this condition have almost no insulin because of a loss of beta cells in the pancreas where insulin is made. Studies show that it's due to an immune reaction (insulin auto antibodies) that destroys the beta-insulin producing cells. The type 2 or adult type (most others have this type) requires oral medications first, but these patients have high blood insulin levels, which is called insulin resistance, which I will explain later. These patients may need added insulin too, if they cannot be controlled.

Just recently, research has led to a greater understanding of diabetes and has even redefined its diagnosis and treatment. It is now defined as having a fasting blood sugar of greater than 100, which is its most common presentation with no symptoms. The secret here, "no symptoms," means that you could have diabetes and not know it unless you had that yearly physical exam and a blood test drawn. For example, it is estimated that with adult diabetes, the patient will have it for seven years before it's discovered.

If symptoms do occur, they would include polyuria, polydipsia, and poly-phagia, which mean increased urine, thirst, and eating, respectively, along with weight loss. Generally these symptoms occur when the blood sugar levels are over 400, which can be very dangerous and lead to diabetic ketoacidosis with coma and death, if not treated. The secret with symptoms is that they can be highly insidious, such as fatigue and visual blurring. The visual blurring occurs because the increased blood sugar levels increase the sugar levels in the eye, which makes it hard to see through, like a cloudy bathroom window.

More recently, research has revealed actual subtypes of adult diabetes. In these patients, fasting blood sugars may be normal, but their postprandial sugars (two hours after eating) are elevated. Normally after you eat, your blood sugars should be under 160, but in these patients, they're greater, and despite having normal fasting blood sugars (less than 100), these patients need to be treated. Also, for many years a fasting blood sugar of under 150 was considered a watch-ful waiting phase, and under 100 was considered normal. Now we know that patients in the 100–150 category need to be treated because their complication rates are also very high. They are called pre diabetes. That means that your doc-tor needs to be aggressive in diagnosis and treatment, and he or she is not just a mean person.

Why is this so important, and why so nit-picking? The monumental secret is that diabetes is not a disease of elevated blood sugars, but a disease of blood vessels. Unless you sugar is over 400, like I said, you probably will not have any symptoms, but during the entire time that blood sugar is elevated—whether postprandial, fasting, or between the 100–150 range—your blood vessels are aging with atherosclerosis. Silently, relentlessly, you are aging like a cancer malignancy!

Family history may be a secret clue as a risk factor, but since diseases may skip generations (your grandparent may have diabetes but not your parent), you might miss it. The most important secret is regulating the blood sugar, which is mandatory, along with having a blood test called the A1C that measures the blood sugar levels over a period of thirty to ninety days, and which is a true indicator of just how good the blood sugar control is. The A1C needs to be between 5 and 6, but the biggest problems overall tend to be weight control, exercise, and diet, and taking the medications properly. Diabetics also need a yearly eye exam by an ophthalmologist to examine their retinas to look for early changes of neovascularization (new blood vessels) that can be treated with a laser to prevent blindness.

The onset of diabetes can be silent (no symptoms), so it takes a real effort on the part of the doctor and patient to confront these problems and treat them effectively over the long term. The secret here with the new entities called prediabetes and postprandial diabetes requires treatment that would include medication (metformin) along with the nutritional secrets such as green-coffee extract, carnosine, blueberry extract, and AMPK (adenoside monophosphate), in addition to weight control and exercise. I might add that the natural remedies work well by themselves, so they need to be considered when the diagnosis is made, and many times will obviate the use of insulin, so that's a good incentive to take them.

As a reminder, it's imperative for you to remember that diabetes is not a disease of blood sugar, but a disease of blood vessels. I can't tell you how important this is, because that means that in a poorly controlled diabetic who is forty years old, for example, he or she will have blood vessels of an eighty-year-old. That's why patients like this have strokes, heart attacks, neuropathies, blindness, and amputations. It's a blood-vessel disease and not a blood sugar disease, which is a well-kept secret and needs to be reiterated. So if you have diabetes without symptoms, the disease is still aging you. Talk about the cost of medicine and treating all these presumed preventive complications! It's astronomical—and a financial malignancy eating at the fabric of medicine.

Finally, there needs to be a physician involved who is equally aggressive and shares these beliefs to spend the time to "git 'er done," like that cable guy says. I hate to say it, but I must: most of the endocrinologists that I see here in Florida undertreat their diabetics and seem to be satisfied with poor control and way-too-high A1C levels. They are not aggressive enough, and it drives me crazy, but of course they have no knowledge of nutrient therapies that can help immensely!

Diet, activity, weight loss, and the use of insulin and oral medications are what are typically used. I require my diabetic patients to check their blood sugar before breakfast, lunch, supper, and bedtime every day. They are to write the numbers down and bring their log in with their next visit so that I can review them. You see, the secret here is that the blood sugar needs to be controlled all day long, not just in the morning, which is a fundamental mistake that many doctors make (by taking fasting blood sugars only).

The nutritional secret is that we can, as mentioned, add blueberries, green-coffee extract, AMPK, and carnosine, which will not only help lower blood sugars, but help abort many of the complications of diabetes. More recently, resveratrol, omega-7 oils, pycnogenol, pomegranate K2, and the omega-3 oils would also be recommended. These nutrients will not only control blood sugars, but will prevent long-term problems with such areas as the eyes, peripheral neuropathies, heart attacks, and strokes.

Here are some of the historical nutritional secrets and their discovery. In 1923, before insulin was discovered by Banting and Best, there was a report in the *American Journal of Medicine* that concluded that bilberry or blueberries were probably the only available treatment that worked for diabetes. It works as an adjunct to standard medical treatment by lowering blood sugar levels and decreasing insulin resistance, which results in better sugar utilization.

Green-coffee extract, because of the chlorogenic acid in it, decreases blood sugar the same way and will also decrease weight. Some studies reported that the chlorogenic acid acted like metformin—a drug that we use from the French lilac—that decreases gluconeogenesis (makes sugar) in the liver through glucose 6-phosphatase and stimulates intracellular AMPK to utilize energy better, which will drop sugar levels in the blood. Its mechanism of action has nothing to do with insulin, which is a good quality to have and, therefore, the patient can avoid hypoglycemia (low blood sugar).

In a study group on green-coffee extract, investigators noted a 17 percent weight loss that would help with obese diabetics. In addition, pomegranate stimulates the PONS receptors (paraoxonase) on the HDL molecules that remove plaque from blood vessels, which reduces the atherosclerosis seen with diabetics. The HDL is like a good taxi in our bloodstream that takes plaque off our vessels and transports them to the dump (the liver) to be metabolized. On the other hand, the LDL molecules are the bad cholesterol (bad taxicabs that bring the lipids to the blood vessels and cause heart attacks), and that's why your LDL blood level must be 60 or less. The EPA (omega-3 oils) and olive oils in essence do the same thing as pomegranate does while reducing triglyceride levels and elevating the "good" HDL levels that reduce the plaque seen in diabetics. K2 removes calcium from blood-vessel walls (where the calcium causes hardening of the arteries) and deposits the calcium in our bones where it belongs, thereby reducing blood-vessel aging and helping prevent osteoporosis.

The omega-7 oils and pycnogenol lower the LDL (bad cholesterol) and raise the HDL (good cholesterol) by improving blood flow and preventing blood starvation to the tissues. You can see the nutrition secret here for using several agents to get maximum effect in diabetics, which treats its root cause and, at the same time, results in patients' using less medication, including insulin.

With the advancing blood-vessel disease in diabetics, we now have realized that tissue aging occurs as a result of AGEs (advanced-glycation end products). The secret here is that AGEs are sugar molecules that hook onto proteins called aldehydes. These aldehydes then inactivate their proteins, like our cellular DNA, which leads to accelerated aging because our cells cannot reproduce themselves effectively. They get old. You can see these end products in people's faces, with the vertical wrinkles around the mouth and wrinkles in general (skin aging). The secret here is that carnosine can prevent this from happening and needs to be given to all diabetics, wrinkles or not. You can think of carnosine as preventing the "wrinkling" of not only your skin, the largest organ of our body, but of all organ systems, even the internal ones.

With diabetics, you may hear the expression *insulin resistance*, which means that the blood insulin levels are high, but the insulin is not working; this occurs almost exclusively with the type 2 diabetics. In type 1, as a comparison, insulin levels are very low and even zero. The insulin resistance in a type 2 is due to many reasons, but obesity, with decreased levels of adiponectin, is probably the most common reason. Normal adipocyte, or small fat, cells make adiponectin that decreases insulin resistance and decreases tumor necrosis factor, which causes generalized body inflammation. Obese adipocytes, or large fat cells, make less adiponectin and increase insulin resistance and increase tumor necrosis factor, which increases body inflammation.

As obesity is treated with weight loss, small adipocytes replace the large ones and secrete more adiponectin, which, in turn, decreases blood sugar levels commensurate with it because there is less insulin resistance. Therefore, weight loss reverses a very bad negative cycle. Also, that large belly seen in many people with diabetes is more than just a visual distraction, with larger pants or dress size, but is a secreting endocrine organ that also secretes estrogen, which causes breast enlargement (gynecomastia) in men and increased breast cancer risk in women.

What this all means is that with diabetes mellitus, we need an early diagnosis, great control of the blood sugar, a normal BMI (weight control), and careful monitoring. If the condition is mild, then nutritional measures may be all that's necessary, but if moderate to severe, medications including the oral agents and insulin will be required.

One last secret: do not be afraid of insulin treatment. It is easy to deliver, comes in dial-up pens that do not require refrigeration, and will lead to better control. There is now a long-acting drug called Tresiba, which works over forty-four hours and offers great control with no hunger, which the other insulins do cause—something called the Somogyi effect. All too often, patients are afraid of the suggestion that insulin will be necessary, which I think comes from a needle fear, or it subconsciously means to the patients that they are doing worse. These concerns could not be further from the truth. As a matter of fact, my diabetics on insulin do better because I can precisely control their blood sugars with the insulin as compared to the oral agents.

In summary, get your physical every year and have your blood checked for diabetes, and also be aggressive in controlling weight, blood sugars, and other risk factors such as elevated lipid (fat) levels and hypertension. I tell my patients that, unless they do these things while feeling no symptoms, the diabetes will "eat them alive," which is a slight overstatement, but is true. Whatever it takes for them to do what is necessary is my strategy, and fright is a good one.

Twelve

THE SECRETS OF THE EYE

*E*ye diseases many times are linked to systemic diseases such as diabetes and hypertension (high blood pressure). Yes, there are many primary diseases of the eyes too, and these need to be understood, but they can be both prevented and treated with nutrients.

The Eye

Since the eye is so intimately involved with diabetes, I thought that we should discuss it next. Diabetes affects the back of the eye (retina) by forming new blood vessels in a process called neovascularization. The vessels need to be found and treated with laser therapy before blindness occurs. These new (neo-) blood vessels are very fragile and break, causing the retinal layers to separate, which leads to blindness. I might add that these processes do not cause any symptoms until it's too late.

Before we go any further, let's review some anatomy of the eye so that we may better understand diseases of the eye. First, the eye has two chambers; the anterior is defined by the cornea (the window of the eye) in front and posteriorly by the lens (the camera lens of the eye). The posterior chamber is defined by the lens anteriorly and the retina posteriorly, where light waves are converted to electrical transmissions to the brain for interpretation.

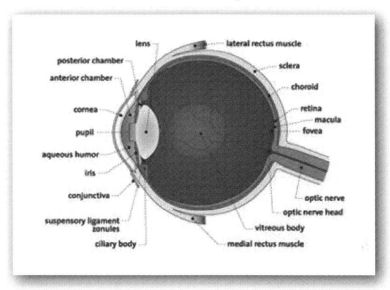

The visual image that we see is processed in a somewhat convoluted way, in that the lateral part is transmitted to the same side of the brain; whereas, the medial part is transmitted to the opposite side of the brain. This occurs because these medial fibers cross over in an area of the brain called the chiasma, which sits just in front of the pituitary. That's why patients with pituitary tumors many times have problems with medial vision but from the opposite side of the brain, as compared to the lateral vision, which is on the same side of the brain. Granted, this is confusing, but unless you are an ophthalmologist or neurologist, it is unimportant.

The most common cause of blindness in the United States is macular degeneration. Since the macula in the retina is responsible for central vision, patients with macular degeneration lose that part of their visual field. Aging, along with the radiation effects of the sun (ultraviolet waves), are the reasons for macular degeneration. This tells us something of the treatment, which is to decrease the effects of the sun by avoiding excessive sun exposure—for example, wearing hats with large brims with sunglasses. A baseball hat alone can decrease ultraviolet exposure to the eye by 60 percent as long as you wear the brim forward and not backward.

There are two types of macular degeneration: the wet type can be treated early with laser, and the dry type is much harder to treat, is unresponsive to laser, and unfortunately is the most common. The secret here is that nutritional therapy with carnosine, vitamin C, beta-carotene, lutein, bilberry (blueberry), lycopene, and zeaxanthins works in preventing and actually treating an established problem. The latter five nutrients have high concentrations of proanthocyanidins, which are nutritious to the retina. Eating foods with high concentrations of these same chemicals will help. They are the fruits and vegetables that have a red color, such as red bell peppers. Studies have shown that 30–60 percent of the macular effects can be aborted or improved. If you remember that the retina is color dependent, you will shop a whole lot differently because we are what we eat.

The lens of the eye is most affected by cataracts or clouding of the lens. These conditions are part of the aging process in all of us, but sun exposure and other risk factors such as diabetes can accelerate it, which may require surgery. Another secret is that if you need surgery, you will have a choice: the old-fashioned procedure that removes only the cataract, which Medicare pays for almost 100 percent; or the new lens-insertion technique that will cost you about $3,000 an eye because Medicare won't pay for it. After the surgery, you should have twenty-twenty vision in both eyes regardless of which surgery you have chosen, but the lens-replacement groups have more complications. So it's your choice in terms of cost and results. Just make sure that the eye doctor gives you one.

Incidentally, the yardstick that I use for my patients is that if you can read the newspaper, then you don't need surgery. The real secret with cataracts is prevention, so avoid excessive sun exposure by wearing hats with large brims and sunglasses, not only for you, but for your children. Carnosine and high doses of vitamin C (2,000–3,000 mg/day) will also help to prevent cataracts. Don't rush to surgery and *never* have both eyes operated on at the same time. Why? Because there are problems with all surgeries, and if both eyes are done and problems occur, you could end up blind.

The retina is king when it comes to eye diseases because of its vulnerability and its importance. It takes the light rays and converts them to brain waves (light waves to nerve and chemical transmission), which are mediated through rods and cones in the retina. This chemical transformation includes not only images, but color too. How remarkable!

You've heard of a retinal detachment, when the layers of the retina separate, which occurs because of aging, hypertension, head trauma, or the diabetic process. The same nutrients and foods that help treat and prevent macular degeneration (such as beta-carotene, lutein, zeaxanthin, blueberries [bilberries], and lycopene) will do the same thing for the retina detachment because the retina is again the major victim. Here again, the secret is that nutrients are much more helpful than any medication, with the exception of a retinal detachment, which requires eye surgery to repair. As a corollary, all diabetics need to be on this regimen to help prevent diabetic blindness as a result of retinal problems. More recently, zinc has been shown to nourish the retina, and I would add it to the regimen.

One more thing, a lesson from history during World War II: the RAF (English Royal Air Force) pilots who fought the Germans took blueberries to help them see better at night. The proanthocyanidins in it enriched the retina, which improved night vision to better help the pilots shoot down German aircraft during the night raids. That was seventy years ago! Therefore, if you are having night-vision problems, take blueberries or blueberry extract.

Thirteen

THE SECRETS OF THE BRAIN

The brain has received a lot of attention because of Alzheimer's disease, as well it should, but we must not forget that there are important new considerations. New concepts on how the brain can grow after being damaged are of the first order to consider, and they need special attention because nutrients play a major role in doing that very thing.

The Brain

The high-command center of our body is the brain (*el Jefe*). Through its sensory system, we analyze what is going on (through pain and sensory receptors), and then the brain commands the body how to react through its motor system (muscles). Our nervous system is broken down into the central nervous system (CNS), which includes the brain itself and the spinal cord, along with the peripheral nervous system, which includes the nerves that go out of our spinal cords into our extremities. This distinction is important because many diseases will only affect the brain or spinal cord, but not both, so depending on the symptoms and our physical findings, we can discern the difference, and thus a diagnosis is easier to make.

I think that most people are aware that the brain is vulnerable to damage because it needs oxygen (O_2) and sugar now, not later, which means that without them for two minutes, damage will occur. Because it is so vulnerable, the brain has a hard covering over it to protect it, called the skull, which makes sense, and that's why we don't wear a helmet when riding a bike or motorcycle! Wrong! The brain, however, in its bony protective helmet (skull) can sustain damage if the skull is traumatized by banging against it, to and fro, in what are called coup and contra-coup injuries. The damaged or bruised brain is called a concussion, which is a now a big deal with football players. Chronic traumatic encephalopathy (CTE) eventually leads to Alzheimer's disease and Parkinsonism. There is now good evidence to suggest that repeated concussions can lead to permanent brain damage later in life. Boxer Muhammad Ali, who died with severe Parkinsonism, is a good example.

Anatomically, arterial blood through the carotid (anterior) and vertebral (posterior) blood vessels are the main highways of blood into the brain, but the carotids are the major vessels. Any disruption of these blood supplies within a short period of time (two minutes) can lead to a transient ischemic attack (TIA), or a stroke. We only use a small part of our brain in regard to memory and thinking (about 10 percent), so there is a large reserve factor when it comes to brain injuries. The one exception is the spinal cord, however, including the brain stem, where there is a very small space surrounded with bone where even small injuries can be catastrophic. The brain stem or upper part of our spinal cords in our neck also includes the autonomic heart and breathing centers that, if damaged, can result in sudden death (neck fractures).

The nervous system works like the electricity in your home, with currents via neurotransmitter chemicals (acetylcholine, serotonin, and dopamine) that are carried through neurons (wires) and across synapses, which are junctions between the wires that act like relay switches. Any disruption of these transmissions, depending on where they are, can affect sensory and motor function. Cancer can affect both the central and peripheral nervous system, but with our CT and MRI scans, the cancers are now easily found if we are suspicious enough. You will be surprised how effective nutrients can be in the prevention and treatment of many nervous-system diseases. Even though there are many mechanisms by which they work, many mechanisms by which they work in combinations, their effects can be enhanced.

I'm sure that if I asked all seniors, "Are you worried about getting Alzheimer's disease?" most would say yes. The same would be true of their families too, because many times they will be the caretakers, spending endless hours and money to care for their elders. If I had asked that same question thirty years ago, however, most people would say no, because then people did not live long enough to get it. That means that since people are living longer, degenerative diseases that affect the elderly, such as Alzheimer's disease, have become very relevant. We just don't see Alzheimer's disease in young people.

Beta-amyloid plaques and tau proteins in the cerebral cortex are the reason why Alzheimer's develops, but how the plaques and proteins form is still an open question. At this point, aging along with oxidative processes are relevant factors. Forgetful behavior is an early symptom in a retrograde manner, which means that recent things are the most problematic. For example, patients with early stage Alzheimer's cannot remember what they ate yesterday but have no trouble with relatives' names or events of the past. The secret is that if the patient knows that he or she is forgetting, then it probably is not Alzheimer's disease.

Aricept and Namenda are helpful, but the overall prognosis is not good, since neither drug will reverse the pathology. The secret here is that now we know that it is the oxidative degenerative process that is the basic pathophysiology (what causes Alzheimer's) that leads to the amyloid plaques and tau proteins, and that nutrients are a big help in not only preventing the problem, but also in treating it. That would include EPA (omega-3 oils), resveratrol, curcumin, pycnogenol, acetylcarnitine, CoQ10, PQQ, phosphatidylserine (PS), and gingko. More recently, with the discovery of brain growth or plasticity, gastrodin from a Chinese orchid, green tea, and magnesium threonate researched by MIT are recommended and also for athletes to prevent the concussive brain injuries. Starting the regimen earlier is best because reversing the oxidative inflammatory process of the beta-amyloid and tau proteins is key before Alzheimer's really gets started.

There is a variant between Alzheimer's disease and Parkinsonism, which is called Lewy body dementia. These patients share symptoms of both but may have hallucinations. This will be my third year in speaking at the West Palm Beach Alzheimer's Disease Society conference, and it always gives me great pleasure in talking about nutrients and how good they are in preventing and treating brain problems.

Strokes, or cerebral vascular accidents (CVA), occur when the brain is deprived of O_2 and/or sugar because of the lack of blood flow to it. The two most common mechanisms are thrombosis, which is the most common, where a plaque and blood clot obstruct the artery within the brain; and a cerebral hemorrhage, which occurs as a result of a congenital aneurysm (like a bubble on a tire) or hypertension (high blood pressure) that results in a "blowout" of the artery. The presenting symptoms are those of a sudden onset of a severe headache, speech impediment, or weakness or paralysis with other mental or physical impairments.

If the symptoms last less than twenty-four hours and resolve, then it is considered a TIA, or transient ischemic attack. TIAs serve as a major red flag or warning, mandating a stat (immediate) MRI and carotid studies with appropriate medication to avoid a future completed stoke.

The secret with all these is prevention, because if you wait for the main event, it could be catastrophic (causing death or paralysis). Controlling blood sugar, blood pressure, lipids, and other risk factors is key, which again mandates that yearly physical exam. Nutrients play a unique role here because they can help correct all these factors, along with neutralizing the free-radical oxidative damage that may be present. The secrets include the EPA omega-3 oils, omega-7 oils, resveratrol, PQQ, olive oil, pomegranate, K2, pycnogenol, branched-chain amino acids, lipoic acid, and acetylcarnitine.

With high blood pressure, the natural secrets are CoQ10, PQQ, taurine, and hawthorn along with standard medications, if necessary. Normalizing the blood pressure is absolutely required, and I might add that hypertension can be present without symptoms for years, which is why that yearly physical is so important. Also, don't depend on the grocery-store scale or mechanical blood pressure machines, because they are notoriously inaccurate. These devices could read out a normal weight and blood pressure when in fact levels are elevated, therefore putting you at risk for a stroke, heart attack, or kidney failure.

As a matter of fact, hypertension is the most common cause of kidney failure. If you want to end up on dialysis, keep letting the grocery store take care of you! With my overly suspicious mind, I could see where the grocery stores would intentionally lower the scale readouts so that people would think that their weight was not elevated and would therefore buy more food! If the scale read high, they would buy less, right?

Parkinsonism

A disease of generally older people with some exceptions (Michael J. Fox), Parkinsonism affects the deep, older areas of the brain where you find decreased levels of dopamine in the substancia nigra (midbrain), which leads to problems with walking (ataxia), tremor, and progressive dementia. Standard medical therapy is quite good in the form of Sinemet and Azilect (dopamine repleters that increase brain dopamine levels), which actually improve symptoms, but more importantly, the progression will stop.

Symptoms include problems with speech, a shuffling gait with less arm swing, a facial expression like staring, and a tremor. Memory loss generally follows with dementia that can be slowly progressive or very progressive.

Here's the secret with Parkinsonism. In using CoQ10 in high doses of up to 900 mg/day, vitamin D (5,000 units a day), and pycnogenol, the progression of the Parkinsonism will stop and improve. PQQ (pyrroquinoline quinone) more recently has been shown to have a synergistic effect (it increases benefit) when used with the CoQ10, so I would advise that you use them in tandem. But here again, early diagnosis and early treatment are critical for better outcomes, so that yearly exam becomes critical.

One more thing: there is a definite relationship of Parkinsonism to volatile organic solvents (VOCs) such as paint solvents, acetone, formaldehyde, and the like, so avoid them at all costs, and think ventilation if you can't avoid using them!

Chronic Fatigue Syndrome

A common malady affecting many organ systems including the brain, chronic fatigue syndrome is a bit unique because it affects both young and old patients. It presents like just like its name: "I'm sleepy and tired all the time." It used to be considered a psychological problem, a neurosis, but now it is believed to be linked to two viruses: the Epstein-Barr (EB) and cytomegaloviruses (CMV), which are both herpes viruses that have short- and long-term considerations.

You may have heard of the Epstein-Barr virus because years ago it was called the infectious mono virus, but more recently it has changed its presentation. I placed this disease here because many times it gets mixed up with neurological diseases (that is, headaches with generalized weakness), and there may be some basis for it to be considered a neurological disease because these organisms can be found in the brain and nerves. To make it worse, these organisms, over a long period of time, have been linked to vascular autoimmune diseases like lupus, scleroderma, or immune suppression, so patients have frequent and severe recurrent infections.

Finally, lymphoma (a lymph-node cancer) may occur years later, so that means that we not only have to make a correct diagnosis, but also treat it and get rid of the organisms. Unfortunately, there are no medications that will get rid of EB/CMV viruses directly, but there is a secret nutrient cocktail that will first stop the viruses from replicating and then get rid of them.

Sometimes patients complain of muscle aches and pains, a variant, along with the extreme fatigue, that is called fibromyalgia. Blood tests in these patients will show an elevation of inflammatory markers (C-reactive proteins and sedimentation rates and elevated viral antibody titers). Generally, the autoantibody blood tests for lupus and the like will become positive later in the course of the disease, with more symptoms of joint pains.

The secret nutrients include fucoidans, lipoic acid, branched-chain amino acids, zinc, and reishi mushrooms with cistanche, all of which will, in combination, increase the body's immune system through immune "T" cells, which rid the body of these unwanted organisms. Within seven to ten days, patients feel better and have more energy. Gradually, over two to three months, the virus should disappear. For these patients with immune-disease findings like a positive

ANA (antinuclear antibody blood test) for lupus, add peony extract and mung bean with HMG Box 1 extract to "cool down" this exaggerated response.

Let me warn you, however, that many doctors consider this chronic fatigue complaint to have no merit and will treat you like a neurotic head case with that serum "porcelain level"—an expression that doctors use for a crackpot—and will dismiss you. If that is your case, find another doctor who is more knowledgeable and sympathetic.

Fibromyalgia

In addition to the chronic fatigue syndrome, there is some evidence that the muscular and nervous systems can be affected as well, which I mentioned earlier. I consider this a variant of the chronic fatigue syndrome with symptoms that include fatigue and tiredness along with muscle and joint aches and pains, which can be very prominent. There is generalized muscle tenderness on exam and perhaps a reduction in reflexes, indicating a peripheral nerve problem, which you see with immune diseases like lupus, polymyositis, and dermatomyositis or from drug side effects seen with statin medications that need to be ruled out.

Lyrica and Neurontin are the most common drugs used, but in my experience, they don't work. I have found that the bundling of nutrients, as mentioned above, with chronic fatigue syndrome will work here also, along with more nutrient anti-inflammatories. The real secret here is that Zyflamend, a Chinese herbal remedy of nine ingredients, along with resveratrol and curcumin and their strong anti-inflammatory actions, is very useful in getting rid of the muscle aches and pains. Here again, many physicians will dismiss you as a nutcase, so my advice would be to find another doctor.

Incidentally, Columbia University has research (published November 7, 2005, in the journal *Nutrition and Cancer*) about Zyflamend in regard to prostate cancer too, and its researchers recommend that if you are at risk (if you are, for example, a Vietnam veteran with Agent Orange exposure or have a father with prostate cancer) or have it, then take Zyflamend. This study's response rates were near 30 percent.

Neuropathy

Diseases of the peripheral nervous system cause numbness and tingling with pain in the extremities (mostly the legs), depending on where the disease process is at work. The secret in dealing with neuropathies is that they need to be diagnosed and treated early and with vigor to avoid motor and sensory loss with possible paralysis.

One example is carpal tunnel syndrome, which occurs in the hands with numbness, tingling, and pain in the palm of the hand. It occurs because the median nerve is being compressed by the wrist ligaments. Steroids, Pennsaid (a rub-on), and anti-inflammatory medication with night braces are used, but the secret is in using nutrients like EPA omega-3 oils, mung bean, curcumin, UC (undenatured collagen), and Zyflamend, which may be a better choice since they are cheap and without side effects.

Risk factors include hypothyroid disease (low thyroid), protein diseases (amyloidosis), and obesity. Men, especially those who use their hands a lot (manual laborers), are at risk, as are people with any of the arthritic diseases. If carpal tunnel is severe enough, laparoscopic surgery will be necessary to relieve the pressure on the tendons and restore normal function, but that is always a last resort. Generally, a hand surgeon will inject the wrist first with steroids, and, if the injection is unsuccessful, then surgery will be done. In addition, weight loss is critical if the patient is overweight, because all the medications in the world will fail unless you take the pressure off the nerve from the fat tissue.

The most common and perhaps the most problematic neuropathy is linked to diabetes. Neuropathies affect the feet, mostly with numbness and pain, so unless the blood sugars are controlled, neuropathy can be devastating. EPA omega-3 oils, omega-7 oils, B-complex vitamins, lipoic acid, pycnogenol, vinpocetine, and huperzine in combination with blood sugar control will first stop the progression and then improve it. New scientific data suggest that the neuropathy results from microvascular (tiny blood vessels) changes, so that's where our emphasis should be. Risk factors like hypertension or lipid problems need to be aggressively sought after and treated, but patients need to understand that treatments will take months to work, so they should be patient. Unfortunately, in my experience, medical therapy with Lyrica and Neurontin has not been effective. By the way, Lyrica is very expensive and poses significant side effects.

Other causes of neuropathies include heavy-metal poisoning (from lead, for example), B12 and B6 vitamin deficiencies, and Lyme disease, which all have to be ruled out. If there is a B deficiency, then B-complex and/or B12 will be used. Heavy-metal poisoning occurs mostly with lead or mercury, and a blood test will help. Lead sources are generally industrial or from paint and mercury, most commonly from vegetarians eating fish that have high mercury levels. The secret here is to find the source and use selenium, vitamin E, and vitamin C to help lower these levels. With the heavy metals, if high enough, blood-chelating agents like EDTA can be used as IV therapy.

Myositis

I put myositis (inflammation of the muscles) in this chapter because the symptoms for it are almost identical to fibromyalgia and chronic fatigue syndrome, with similarities to neuropathies. Myositis means inflammation of the muscles (striated ones) that power our mobility—therefore, our arms and legs. There are two autoimmune diseases (that make abnormal antibodies to muscles) called polymyositis and dermatomyositis (muscle pain with a rash), in which autoantibodies are being made against one's own muscles, which can cause muscle pain, weakness, and fatigue. Because of the muscle inflammation, muscles are very weak, and patients have problems walking and even getting off the toilet or out of a chair.

When these symptoms occur, your doctor also needs to rule out that other medications being taken could be causing problems. Specifically, statins (cholesterol medication) have to be discontinued.

Myasthenia gravis may be mixed up with the muscle pain and weakness, but with myasthenia the muscle weakness generally occurs later in the day. Patients feel normal in the morning. On physical exam, just squeezing the muscles reproduces the pain, thereby separating it from joint pain and arthritis. Blood tests measuring muscle enzymes and antibodies to the muscles are generally diagnostic (positive).

Treatment using steroids will be helpful, but steroids over a long period of time can lead to toxicity like diabetes, fluid retention, cataracts, and osteoporosis, so the secret with the nutrients is that they come to the rescue. Anti-inflammatories like Zyflamend along with carnitine, branched-chain amino acids, mung bean extract, peony, lipoic acid, curcumin, and resveratrol will help immeasurably. The inflammatory laboratory parameters in the blood, such as sed rate, CRP, and proinflammate levels (tumor necrosis factor, interleukins), will go down. Finally, many times standard medications in combination with these nutrients will be helpful and, at the very least, require less medication with less expense.

Multiple Sclerosis (MS)

This is truly a disease of the nervous system, both central and peripheral, but because of the nature of its symptoms, multiple sclerosis may be confused with muscle diseases. MS is an autoimmune disease of the central and peripheral nervous system in which autoantibodies attack the outer lining of nerves, called myelin, resulting in nerve damage, which leads to the symptoms. It's believed that an underlying virus may be the culprit, but as of today, we don't know for sure.

MS is generally found in women in their twenties and thirties. Intermittent neurological symptoms (symptoms that come and go) are key and can manifest as simple muscle weakness or even visual loss. Blood tests, an MRI, x-rays, spinal taps, and a complete neurological exam will be necessary to make a diagnosis, and the medical therapy would include steroids and immune-suppressing medications along with nutrients.

Nutrients would include Zyflamend, lipoic acid, resveratrol, mung bean, peony, B-complex, huperzine, phosphatidylserine (PS), and curcumin, which are all anti-inflammatory, along with beta-carotene, fucoidans, zinc, and reishi mushroom/cistanche extracts, which are all antiviral. The latter increase T-cell levels, which will kill the virus. Since none of these have been investigated, only common sense tells me that they may be helpful, but I need to stress, however, that they are only secondary to the standard medications that come first.

Guillain-Barre Syndrome

This disease of the peripheral and central nervous system starts out with a respiratory infection that many times is very mild and unnoticed (cough, low-grade fever, running nose, for example), but within two to three weeks, the disease is associated with an ascending (feet first) paralysis. Numbness and weakness in the feet progresses up the legs and into the abdomen and chest area, followed by motor loss and paralysis. If the paralysis is high enough, respiratory function is decreased (the patient can't breathe), and the patient could suffocate, so at this point patients have to be put on ventilators to survive. It's believed to be due to an immune reaction to a virus that has gone "astray" and is now affecting the nervous system through antibody production. We see this currently with the Zika virus outbreak, which is a risk factor for both men and women. Nutrient anti-inflammatories like curcumin, resveratrol, Zyflamend, and HMG Box 1, a cytokine inhibiter from mung beans may be of some help.

Fourteen

THE SECRETS OF CANCER

When Richard Nixon was president, he announced a war on cancer and pledged billions of dollars in research to discover its cause and cure, but the cure never happened, even though the money was spent. The reason why was that we did not have the research ability to find cures, but today we do. Let's take a closer look at how nutrients can play a major role in cancer prevention and treatment.

There are no other words that a patient could be told in a doctor's office that produce more fear than "You have cancer." Being a cancer survivor myself and having treated hundreds of people over the last thirty years with cancer, I can tell you that when you're the one with cancer, the disease has a whole different meaning. Immediately it leaves you with a consciousness of your own mortality, along with loneliness, fear, and emptiness that does not go away.

Having a license to carry a concealed weapon—that feeling of empowerment—is just the opposite; you really do feel alone when you have cancer. Ask yourself if you have ever thought about a predetermined death, and that's exactly what the situation is. My guess would be that if you did, it would change your life or at least your outlook and values; like that country song says, "Live your life like you're dying." The worst part about it is that because cancer can recur, it never goes away—a haunting that can undermine everything.

There are two types of cancers: solid tumors and hematogenous cancer, which include the blood and lymph. Why they occur is still being heavily investigated, but we do have some of the answers. Many tumors are genetic in nature. You are born with "cancer gates" or "preloaded genes" that are opened with triggers like viruses, smoking, chemical exposures, and free radicals (oxidation).

Cancer can also occur when the DNA in our cells becomes damaged. Radiation exposure is a good example of what can damage our DNA; this radiation can come from sun exposure (ultraviolet radiation) or electromagnetic fields (EMF) associated with cell phones, computers, routers, Wi-Fi, and many other electronic devices.

There is also mounting evidence that perhaps the most common denominator of cancer is chronic inflammation. There are many examples of this, such as esophagitis (inflammation of the esophagus from reflux) and cancer of the esophagus, inflammatory colitis (ulcerative colitis) and colon cancer, and finally, chronic inflammation of the gallbladder and cancer of the gallbladder. Directly related to this is that certain other conditions can lead to cancer, such as colon polyps, which can lead to colon cancer. It's estimated that 85 percent of colon cancers start as polyps, so that's why they need to be found and removed. Finally, we also know that certain deficiencies can lead to cancer, like B12/folic acid and pernicious anemia especially, which has been directly linked to cancer of the stomach because of faulty DNA.

These are just a few of the mechanisms that we know of that lead to cancer, but there are other cancers that just happen, like mine. I had none of these predispositions, but yet there it was. I was lucky because, as a physician, I knew how very insidious symptoms can be with cancer, and I did the appropriate tests.

My surgery at Long Island Jewish Hospital leads us to another important consideration. Why would a Florida resident go to New York for surgery? The answer is that my particular cancer was best done laparoscopically, and the best place for that was in New York. The surgeon there, Dr. Louis Kavouse, pioneered laparoscopic kidney surgery, so he was the best in my opinion, which is precisely what you need to ask yourself if you are told that you have cancer. Where the best place to be is treated both medically and surgically?

Dr. Kavouse did my surgery, in which he removed 20 percent of my left kidney, on Friday, and I returned to work the following Monday. After five years, I am cancer-free, but even though I am cancer-free now, I must admit that there is still an unsettling feeling that it may recur. I would be remiss if I did not thank Dr. Kavouse publicly, and I would highly recommend him for anyone who has a urinary-tract problem that may need surgery. I also want to thank the Long Island Jewish Hospital for their great care and concern for me.

One last thing: if you have had cancer once, you will be at risk for another type of cancer—that is, you will be at a higher risk than a noncancerous patient—so stay vigilant, get that physical every year, and don't take your fortunate recovery as the end.

Before we discuss the specific cancers and how to deal with them, we need to discuss a strategy. Like many sports, a good offense is a good defense, and cancer is no different, in my opinion. That defense would include a good physical exam every year where considerations are also made for family history and lifestyle (smoking, drinking, and alcohol). For example, if the exam is completely normal, but there is a family history of cancer of the breast or prostate, then more tests may be necessary in those areas.

Don't let me forget, however, to say that total-body CT scans or echocardiogram/Doppler studies done in a strip-mall parking lot as a screen are a waste of time and money. Ask yourself why these tests are being done, who is reading them (how competent he or she is), and what evidence there is that any of these tests will help you prevent cancer or survive longer. Even worse, if they tell you that the tests are normal, then you will not get what really is necessary, like a complete physical exam to find that hidden cancer early enough for it to be curable. Incidentally, you will receive a massive amount of radiation, which puts you at risk for cancer—the very thing you are trying to prevent and diagnose.

A good history and physical exam every year needs to be done, but if the history and physical find something abnormal, then generally other tests are done and a closer follow-up is mandated. In summary, this format is the secret in preventing and treating cancers, and it works. I am a case in point.

The next secret is that if a cancer is found, then it has to be staged with a cell type and degree of spread. This will determine what treatment is indicated and a prognosis, so ask your doctor what the cell type is and what the stage of spread is. This information is the secret to prognosis. Stay informed and make sure you know your prognosis and receive the best treatment that you can get.

That's why I advise patients not to get the cheap insurance plans, because when the specter of cancer does raise its head, I can get patients with better plans the tests they need now—not in three months. I can have patients see the best doctors without the interference of the insurance companies saying that they need approval first and that then only approve doctors in their network.

Let me give you one case in point. A few months ago, a patient of mine on a cheap insurance plan came to me with a headache. It took me two to three weeks of preapproval arguing to get the MRI imaging of the brain that was necessary to make a diagnosis. When a brain tumor was found, it took me another two months to find a neurosurgeon to do the procedure. To make matters worse, in my opinion, this neurosurgeon wasn't even the best qualified. Would you like to be in that situation with a brain tumor? I wouldn't! Whether it's a kidney tumor, which is what I had, or a brain tumor, I want the *best*!

Lung Cancer

Lung cancer is a good place to begin a discussion of cancer because it is the most common cancer we see here in the United States. Adenocarcinoma is the most common cell type. The first secret is that smoking is the most important risk factor, so the patient's history is imperative to know, because if the patient is a smoker or has a family member with cancer of the lung, then a more aggressive diagnostic approach is necessary. I will order every year a CT scan with contrast of the lung in a smoker to hopefully find a small lesion that cannot be seen on a routine chest x-ray. One of the secrets in curing cancer is to find it before it has spread, and this imaging strategy makes sense. When you stop to think about it, a proactive (before-it-happens) approach is also much cheaper on the health-care system, which is a concern for everyone.

A 1990s study at the University of Arizona measured the effects of selenium in preventing skin cancer and concluded that selenium decreased significantly the rate of cancer of the lung, but did nothing for skin cancer, however. Some irony! If you believe that chronic inflammation of the lungs from smoking may be a factor, and I think it is, then a cocktail of antioxidants would also be indicated for preventing lung cancer, especially if you are at risk. That's the second secret.

Besides smoking, other inflammatory conditions of the lung such as chronic bronchitis, bronchiectasis, and gastroesophageal reflux (GERD) may also predispose someone to cancer. Therefore, in my opinion, there are other considerations for antioxidant therapy that would include curcumin, resveratrol, quercetin, mung bean, glutathione/cysteine, EPA, olive oil, andrographia, and pycnogenol, which will all decrease the inflammation. Adding B12, beta-carotene, and folic acid may also help repair the DNA of the lung cells. Again, the secret is to spread the nutrients out over the course of the day (grazing) and for perpetuity (over a long period of time) along with *no smoking*. Finally, there is a new medication called Daliresp that does the same thing in reducing inflammation of the lung. It's a nice addition, but it's expensive.

Breast Cancer

Breast cancer, pound for pound, has more secret misinformation than "Carter's Little Liver Pills". Several years ago, it was reported that estrogen could cause breast cancer, and then it was progesterone. Most recently, it's back to estrogen as a cause, but only estrogen at higher doses and over a ten-year period of time. What next? It's like testosterone with prostate cancer: first it caused prostate cancer, but now it prevents cancer of the prostate. How can we be so wrong?

Like most early cancers, the most common symptoms of breast cancer are no symptoms, and that's why that yearly breast exam and mammogram are so important. Just as an aside, if there is any doubt in regard to the mammogram, get a breast MRI, which is the definitive "gold standard" test for breast cancer.

With breast cancer, the family history is also very important, since the cancer carries a large risk for any female child. There are two types of breast cancer: (1) type 1, or alpha ER, has been linked to breast, ovarian, endometrial (uterus), and colon cancer and is influenced by female hormones; and (2) type 2, or beta ER, is not influenced by female hormones and is inactivated by soy, which acts like an antiestrogen by filling and blocking the receptors.

As part and parcel of my philosophy of an early diagnosis and treatment for a better survival, if there is a family history of breast cancer, I recommend a breast exam and digital mammogram starting at the age of twenty-five. The reason is that I have personally taken care of two women with cancer of the breast in their late twenties, and both died before the age of thirty. They both had family histories of breast cancer, and, like prostate cancer, the younger you are when you get it, the more aggressive the cancer becomes.

If there is no family history, however, you're looking at a yearly breast exam and mammogram after the age of forty. The diagnosis and prognosis will depend on the cell type and degree of spread, so that needs to be established and understood. Finally, that leads us to the secret of preventing and treating cancer of the breast with nutrients, but before we go further, however, I need to review some data.

Over the past few years, genetic testing has become available, and with it a better way to take care of people. With it also has come a lot of misinformation, mainly from likely sources such as TV and movie actresses. BRCA1 and BRCA2 genes, when they mutate, put women at risk for not only breast cancer but ovarian, uterine, and pancreatic cancers. If you are a woman with a family history (your mother has it) of breast cancer or the other types too, then testing for these genes is an option. I will not test for them unless a clear plan is agreed upon by the patient and family—an agreement about what the patient will do if the genetic testing is positive.

In my experience, there is nothing worse than to have a patient who is BRCA gene positive without a clear path in what to do. With the Angelina Jolie issue and her breast cancer risk, of course, it was blown way out of proportion either by her publicist or the media, or both, but there are several options: One, do nothing and get good exams every six months, including x-rays and mammograms (MRIs), and treat with nutrients. Option two is prophylactic treatment with tamoxifen and nutrients like soy protein, green tea, and indole-3-carbinol. Third is prophylactic bilateral breast-removal surgery, but the breast cancer risk is only decreased by 90 percent. You cannot remove all the breast tissue, so the patient will not be 100 percent risk-free.

Just to give you an idea, if you are gene positive, your risk for breast cancer is 60 percent, and ovarian cancer risk is about 40 percent, so it is not a 100 percent test. Far from it! Another consideration is that the BRCA gene test is expensive, and many insurance plans will not pay for it, so check with your plan before it is done so as to avoid a giant lab bill.

As long as I'm on the subject of breast cancer, I will touch on some medical misinformation. For years and still today, I hear my colleagues tell their patients to not take any nutrients when it comes to breast cancer, because taking them won't help and it can make the cancer worse. This could not be any further from the truth.

First, all the epidemiological studies tell us that women from Southeast Asia have a much lower incidence of breast cancer than we do, yet they consume large quantities of green tea and soy protein. Second, the chemicals in soy and green tea only affect type 2 or the beta receptors, not type 1 that is associated with the cancer propagation. These nutrients are the ones that decrease the cancer effects with receptor blocking and rearranging of hormone levels to make them less cancer-driven. It's hard for me to understand these doctors' position when the nutrients work just like the estrogen-blocker drug tamoxifen that they recommend!

Can you see the inconsistency here? Of course, by denying women these natural alternatives, doctors are denying their patients treatment, which drives me crazy. This is not to say that women with either the risk or the cancer should *only* be treated with nutrients. Remember also that breast cancer, like prostate cancers and lymphoma, can recur years later (ten to fifteen years later), so the five-year cure rates do not apply.

The secret here is a bimodal attack of the problem, preferably in prevention, but with constant monitoring under a doctor's direction because when a patient's combined guard is down, that's when cancer will recur with a vengeance. Generally, the second time around, cancer is much harder to treat.

In summary, for years epidemiological studies have told us that women from Southeast Asia live longer than American women and have less breast cancer, even though they smoke considerably more in Asian countries. It's believed that their soy protein and green-tea ingestion are the reasons for the lower rates of breast cancer. If these nutrients are linked, then how do these cultural differences work in preventing the cancer and increasing life span?

It's believed that the isoflavones in soy (genisten, daidzein, and equol) and the polyphenols in the green tea (EGCG, epigallocatechin gallate) act like an antiestrogen in premenstrual women by filling up the estrogen receptors and thereby preventing an estrogen-driven cancer effect. After menopause, the polyphenols the receptors and act like estrogen by exerting its positive effects, and in addition they maintain an increased ratio of estrone (weak estrogen) to estradiol (strong estrogen), thereby decreasing untoward effects of the stronger estradiol. Lastly, it turns out that I3C, or indole-3-carbinol, has the same effect as green tea and soy.

Therefore, I recommend for breast and prostate cancer patients that EPA (anti-inflammatory), green tea, soy, and indole-3-carbinol be used to prevent and treat the cancer in conjunction with the standard medical, surgical, and radiation therapies. The EPA helps remove any NFkB (nuclear factor kappa beta), with its anti-inflammatory effects and proresolution molecules. As an addendum, if there is a strong family history of breast cancer, genetic testing may be indicated, and I would recommend the same nutritional cocktail be used as prevention.

I need to warn you, however, that the medical community is not aware of this data or has rejected it and may tell you that the nutrients, soy, green tea, and 13C may even cause cancer of the breast. To allay your fears, however, the Mayo Clinic did a meta-analysis of fourteen studies and found that soy is not linked to breast cancer in any way, shape, or form.

Prostate Cancer

It's hard to believe, but prostate cancer in many ways emulates breast cancer, and as a result I call them the brother-sister tumors. Prostate cancer was thought to be testosterone driven (testosterone caused it), but now we know that *low* testosterone levels actually can cause prostate cancer. It too is linked to a family history, and "it too," if encountered early, tends to be an aggressive tumor. "It too," like breast cancer, affects more men later in life, but we are seeing more and more prostate cancer early (in men forty to fifty years of age).

There may be no symptoms, so that's why that yearly exam, including a rectal exam (ouch)—yes, a rectal exam—is so important. Prostate cancer has been definitely causally linked to Agent Orange, which causes leukemia too, so if you are a Vietnam veteran, monitor yourself carefully. The presenting symptoms of prostate cancer are those of urinary outlet obstruction with frequent urination during the day and night (nocturia) with perhaps hematuria (bloody urine), but most times there are no symptoms. Benign prostatic hypertrophy (BPH) presents the same way, so symptoms will not differentiate between the two, and BPH is not a malignant condition.

A rectal exam and a PSA "prostatic specific antigen", blood test can be helpful but not foolproof, since a normal PSA does not rule out cancer. It's also true that if the PSA is elevated, it does not rule in cancer of the prostate, and a biopsy may be necessary for confirmation. The secret here is that nutritional therapy may be a major player in preventing cancer and treating BPH—and a useful adjunct with therapy for whatever the root cause is.

Columbia University a few years ago studied Zyflamend, a Chinese herbal remedy, and concluded that if you were at risk for cancer of the prostate or had cancer, it should be prescribed. It's a blend of nine herbs that have, for the most part, anti-COX-2 (cyclooxygenase-2) activity, which has anti-inflammatory effects. There is that inflammation again!

The other secret nutrients are EPA omega-3 oils, saw palmetto, soy, lycopene, I3C, selenium, beta sitosterol, and curcumin. In my patients, I have seen dramatic drops in their PSA levels along with no recurrences of the cancer, which have been sustained for years with this combination. In my previous book, *Fountain of Youth: Making Sense of Vitamins, Minerals, Supplements, and Herbs*, I documented a man with cancer of the prostate with PSA levels of 15 who is still cancer-free after eight years, with a current PSA level of 5, on this regimen.

Again I urge that the nutritional therapies be used side-by-side with the standard medical therapies to maximize their effects. A family history of prostate cancer or exposure to Agent Orange, in my opinion, mandates an aggressive prevention mode of a prostate exam every six months with a PSA level starting at the age of thirty. I tend to be aggressive to prevent and not so aggressive with the treatment, because I would rather prevent. It's a simple premise that I use with all diseases: know the risk factors, find them, and get rid of them early to avoid the problem.

Cancer of the Pancreas

Cancer of the pancreas is not a good cancer to have because, when symptoms occur, generally it has metastasized or spread. Symptoms include epigastric (upper abdominal) pain that radiates into the back (many times straight through), with weight loss.

We are seeing an increase in incidence, and we don't understand why, but it's my guess that modern electronics with the radiation that they emit from their magnetic fields could be the reason why. Other risk factors include diabetes, increased alcohol consumption, recurrent pancreatitis, and heavy-metal exposures. In my opinion and as an aside, laptops, cell phones in our pockets, routers, Wi-Fi, and other electronics may have had something to do with Steve Jobs's pancreatic cancer and death, but this is only conjecture.

Generally, a CT scan of the abdomen will make the diagnosis, and then surgery will be decided on. Drug and radiation therapies are not that effective once a diagnosis is made, with the overall survival measured in months. The secret—a well-kept one—is that three nutrients may help to prevent and treat it, with the main one being GLA (gamma linoleic acid). At the Mayo Clinic, Dr. Ruth Lupu, in the laboratory, found that GLA kills pancreatic cancer cells up to 85 percent, which includes gamma linoleic acid (GLA), curcumin, and soy, which should be used in therapeutic doses.

Another, more recent secret here is that curcumin may help because of its anti-inflammatory benefits by decreasing the incidence of the cancer and may help with its treatment, so I will add this to the regimen and hope that the preliminary data will be substantiated. Finally, if you are at risk for cancer of the pancreas because of increased alcohol intake, family history, or diabetes, take this nutrient regimen.

Liver Cancer (Hepatoma)

Although rare, liver cancer does occur, especially in the context of certain diseases. The cancer may be multicentric (occur at more than one site) and curable if found early, so it needs to be looked for especially in patients at risk with hepatitis C, alcoholics, and those with other chronic inflammatory conditions of the liver like fatty infiltration (NAFLD, nonalcoholic fatty liver disease) or liver fluke infestations (Chinese).

Clues to any of these would be a history of upper-right-quadrant pain or drug use going back even twenty to thirty years, living or visiting China, liver enlargement, and liver-enzyme blood tests that stay elevated. If that is the case, a liver biopsy and a CT scan would be definitive.

Diagnostically, your doctor may use an alpha-fetoprotein blood test to diagnose and also follow you if you have hepatitis C, which I do routinely. Since hepatitis C patients are at risk, any rise in the level could indicate malignant transformation.

The secret here is that nutrients may be of help, although at this point, the study data are lacking. Again, anti-inflammatory nutrients seem reasonable and would include silymarin, andrographia, and resveratrol with pterostilbene, curcumin, and quercetin. Silymarin here is the most effective, and with the newer brands, tissue levels are much higher, making it more effective. Therefore, don't buy the cheap one! Resveratrol and andrographia affect both sides of the genetic process by up-regulating the positive effects of inflammation and down-regulating the genes that cause long-term inflammatory cancer risks such as tumor necrosis factor and interleukins. More and more, therapies are being directed to genetic manipulation and immune anti-inflammation tactics like this.

Finally, not drinking alcohol is mandatory, along with medical treatment for the hepatitis C virus with Harvoni, and of course appropriate medical therapies for any other associated diseases are recommended. This new drug, Harvoni, has cure rates of 90 percent over three months, and that is astounding, but the one pill a day costs about $4,000 per month. Measured, however, against the other not-so-effective therapies and the death rates along with all their health expenses, we all save a lot of money with the new drug.

Gastrointestinal Tumors

Tumors of the gastrointestinal tract are generally noted by their geography. Also, for example, esophagus, stomach, pancreas, liver (discussed already), and colon-rectal tumors are almost all a result of chronic inflammation. Therefore, the key is to diagnose the inflammation problems early and treat and get rid of the cancer, along with close monitoring of the patient. Why? Preventing cancer is more preferable than treating it. Sound familiar?

Esophagus

Chronic inflammation of the lower esophagus is called esophagitis, and it is most commonly due to GERD (gastroesophageal reflux), which presents with burning in the epigastric (upper-abdomen) area, with radiation up into the chest. It may be associated with hoarseness, cough, or dysphasia (problems with swallowing of food or liquids). It can be treated medically and diagnosed with endoscopy where biopsies may be confirmatory.

If on biopsy, however, Barrett's esophagitis is found, special attention is necessary, and intensive therapy should be recommended since it is a premalignant finding. If necessary, ablation techniques are available to cure the problem once and for all if the medical therapy fails.

The secret here is that along with standard medical therapy with Prilosec and Protonix, or any other reflux medications, green tea extracts can help immensely to abort the inflammation and perhaps prevent the cancer. But if it persists, then endoscopic (scope) ablation is done to kill potential cancer cells. Again, people from Southeast Asia have a decreased incidence of this cancer as compared to us, and green tea is probably the answer. The EGCG (epigallocatechin gallate), a polyphenol in the tea, is extremely anti-inflammatory on the

GI tract, but it has to be concentrated because drinking just the tea would take three to five cups to reach therapeutic levels. Resveratrol, pterostilbene, and curcumin may be useful add-ons and will certainly not hurt because of their anti-inflammatory and anticancer properties. They, in review, decrease NFkB, an inflammatory-related chemical that over time acts as a DNA/chromosome transcriptor and can change the cells into malignant ones.

Stomach Cancer

Stomach cancer has been linked to four things: H. pylori, bacteria responsible for ulcerations (chronic inflammation); pernicious anemia; chronic inflammation not related to H. pylori from ongoing ulcer disease; and ingested chemical exposures. The symptoms are those of upper-abdominal pain and burning that keeps recurring despite medical therapy. The pain does not respond readily to medications, tends to get worse, is associated with weight loss, and is exacerbated with food.

Treatment includes abstinence from aspirin, alcohol, caffeine, and smoking because all of these will exacerbate the problems. Patients should take acid-lowering agents like Protonix and Prilosec. Upper endoscopy will make the diagnosis, and a biopsy will reveal the bacteria and whether cancer is present.

Pernicious anemia, or low B12 levels, is associated with achlorhydria (low acid levels in the stomach), which has been associated with cancer of the stomach. The anemia is macrocytic (large cells), along with low B12 levels and antibodies to parietal cells and intrinsic factor, which are blood tests that are definitive for the diagnosis. Vegetarians will become B12 deficient, so that history will be important.

In stomach cancer, prevention is really key because medical therapy for the cancer itself is not so good. Surgical resection, chemotherapy, and radiation, along with antibiotics if the pylori bacteria are present, tend to be only palliative. The one exception, however, is H. pylori in the ulcer phase (early), where antibiotics can be curative for the cancer. Green tea and licorice (European type) called DGL, which stands for deglycyrrhized licorice, along with EPA (omega-3 oils), cranberry extract, and especially olive oil (2 ounces three times a day), will help to rid the body of inflammation and the H. pylori bacteria, so I would recommend this regimen for prevention and therapy. The secret, like for most GI tumors, is prevention and diligence in following these patients carefully along with antioxidant and nutrient therapy.

Colon Cancer

The first secret is that colon cancer may be preventable in most cases, if certain guidelines are followed. A comprehensive exam every year with a rectal exam and stools tested for blood (hema-test) is a must for everyone, but a history of colon cancer in the family, inflammatory colitis, or a history of night work are the red flags that should be raised since they are all risk factors for colon cancer. The latter has been shown to be a risk factor since night workers do not get appropriate melatonin release, and with that the risk goes up by 30 percent.

Finally, it is now recommended that everyone over the age of fifty should have a onetime colonoscopy for surveillance purposes. That yearly physical should include a rectal exam and a stool test for occult blood. Some experts even recommend a yearly flexible sigmoid exam that can be done in the office, but that is debatable.

Symptoms would include rectal bleeding or any change in bowl habits (loose to constipation or vice versa), with a colonoscopy being the diagnostic test of choice, which will not only identify any suspicious lesions, but will allow the doctor to biopsy or remove them at the time of the exam. It is estimated that 85 percent of all colon cancers come from polyps, so if polyps are found, they need to be removed, and repeat colonoscopies will be in order.

The blood test CEA (carcinoembryonic antigen) may be helpful, but it may give false positive (high levels with no cancer) and negative results (with colon cancer present). Even smoking without cancer of the colon will elevate the CEA blood levels. Patients with inflammatory bowel disease such as ulcerative colitis or familial polyposis will also need surveillance colonoscopies because of their increased risk for colon cancer.

With colon cancer, the degree of spread or staging is of paramount importance. Surgical removal, radiation, and chemotherapy may help, but the stage of the cancer at the time of diagnosis will tell you the ultimate prognosis. The secret is again in prevention and knowing that any associated inflammation will increase risk.

Therefore, EPA, olive oil, B12, folic acid, mung bean, resveratrol, PQQ (pyrroloquinoline quinone), and curcumin should be used on anyone at risk. The latter three especially interrupt NFkB. or nuclear factor kappa beta, which acts as an intermediary in the inflammatory process. Yes, even the standard practice of medicine recommends many of these nutrients as a standard medical therapy (can you believe that?). You could even make a case for using this same regimen if the CEA is elevated in and by itself. Finally, apple skins (which have phloridzin in them) and wheat grass (which increases butyrate levels in the colon) decrease polyp and cancer formation. Recently garbanzo beans, (chickpeas) with their resistant starches, amylose and raffinose also create butyrate with the same effect.

Another, more recent secret in preventing colon cancer is based on an old study that concluded that eating broccoli prevented colon cancer. At first, beta-carotene was thought to be the good guy, but now we know that the mechanism of action is due to the apigenin, BITC (beta isothiocyanate), sulforaphane, apple-based quercetin, and Malus sieversii in broccoli.

Lastly, apigenin, according to Harvard researchers, may be the only true cancer preventer because it decreases the inflammation of any tissue in question. Sound familiar? BITC has several mechanisms, including increasing apoptosis, which kills cancer cells; forming butyrate that stabilizes the DNA of the colon-lining cells; and inhibiting cancer cell growth. Finally, sulforaphane inhibits cancer stem cells, while the apple extract, quercetin, decreases inflammation. I call this cocktail that I have personally created the "colonic mojito." Take this mojito even with the risk factors previously mentioned.

Fifteen

THE SECRETS OF THE MUSCULOSKELETAL SYSTEM

*O*ur mobility is dependent on not only skeletal muscles, but also the nerves that innervated them and tell them what to do. A highly coordinated system that seems on the surface rather simple turns out to be complex. Like all other areas of the body, the key is to decipher what is wrong and then apply the cure. Here, nutrients play a big role.

Musculoskeletal System

I have already discussed part of this category with our discussion of skeletal muscle and myositis (inflammation of muscles), which leaves only the joints, but this affects so many people that it is of great importance. There are basically two types of joint diseases: rheumatoid and osteoarthritis.

Rheumatoid is an immune reaction to our joints, more specifically to the synovial linings (outer capsule), which causes pain and swelling especially in the morning with eventual joint destruction and deformity.

Osteoarthritis, on the other hand, is the wear-and-tear type of arthritis that affects all our joints (mostly weight-bearing ones), including our spine. When osteoarthritis affects the spine, it sometimes is referred to as spondylitis (inflammation) or spinal stenosis (scarring and narrowing of the cord).

Chronic inflammation (that word again) is the basic pathophysiology in both cases, but there is more to it. In both cases, the joint collagen becomes exposed—one from the immune reaction and the other from the physical rubbing—but, regardless, it is the underlying, exposed collagen that leads to the inflammatory reaction. Therefore, they share a common denominator and also share some of the same treatments.

For example, undenatured collagen is now available, which basically desensitizes the joint areas and creates blocking antibodies generated through the gastrointestinal tract that then abort the immune reaction. It dials down the T cells that cause the inflammation. In addition, it's interesting that investigators, when looking for an allergen that would be identical to human collagen, found it in chickens. This collagen was almost identical chemically but also similar in its three-dimensional configuration (stoichiometrically), which made it a perfect oral agent, called undenatured collagen (UC).

This is the *true* secret in arthritis management. Standard medical care is mostly anti-inflammatory and usually includes nonsteroidal analgesics, steroids, and occasionally immune suppressive drugs (for the rheumatoid type), and they work.

There is one last secret. In osteoarthritis, the cartilage in the joint space gets worn down, decreasing the joint space and causing the bones to rub on each other and, therefore, making the arthritis worse. Glucosamine with MSM (methylsulfonylmethane) and condroitin not only decrease joint inflammation but also increase cartilage growth and create a joint lubricant to "oil" the joint. In regard to lubrication, there is an injectable drug called Hyalgan that does the same thing, but after six injections, it will only last six months, and it's very expensive.

Lastly, Zyflamend, a Chinese herbal remedy, with its COX-2 activity that I talked about before, may be added and can be very effective especially for patients who cannot tolerate standard medication. In summary, undenatured collagen extract and Zyflamend are used in both types of arthritis to decrease inflammation, while glucosamine and MSM are used in osteoarthritis to increase the joint space, decrease bone-on-bone contact, and lubricate. The glucosamine must be 1,500 mg per day, so check the dose carefully. It can take three months to start working, so be patient. Also, if you have an allergy to seafood or iodine, it's advised that you not take it because it comes from seashells.

In discussing the musculoskeletal system, we must not forget the bones themselves. The most important primary bone disease is osteoporosis, which is believed to start developing during our teenage years and affects women in much greater numbers: nine women to every man. That means, of course, that it can affect men too, so don't forget it.

Over the years, we lose calcium from our bone matrix, not the cortex, which weakens the bone and causes pathological fractures and forward stooping. Unfortunately, as a result, we will all lose about two to three inches of height as we get older, and this is the reason why—along with gravity, of course. That means that if you are short to begin with, you have more to lose, so get screened for osteoporosis and start therapy early.

A diagnosis can be made with a DEXA scan, which measures matrix calcium and should be done on all women over the age of fifty every two years—and younger women if there is a family history. The medical recommendations include 1,500 mg of calcium daily (not calcium carbonate), 5,000 IU/day of vitamin D3, and an etidronate medication (like Fosamax), if the scan shows, in fact, osteoporosis.

But the real secret here is vitamin K2. Incidentally, if the scan only shows osteopenia, which is an abnormally low bone density but not bad enough to be osteoporosis, then only the calcium and vitamin D are recommended. Vitamin K2 takes calcium from our blood vessels and puts it back into our bones, so you get a double benefit by decreasing hardening of the arteries (atherosclerosis) and strengthening your bones at the same time. It works through three chemicals—bone Morphogenic protein Z, matrix GLA, and osteopontin—which are responsible for the shift.

Another secret is that I will use the K2 with pomegranate and EPA in patients with carotid disease who may have advancing atherosclerosis. That's why carotid Doppler studies are of benefit and should be done on all patients with risk factors for cardiovascular disease (such as increased lipids, diabetes, high blood pressure, or a family history of arteriosclerotic heart disease). I have seen "beyond belief" improvement in carotid artery disease with this regimen, and patients have thus avoided surgery and possible stroke or death. The plaque in the artery actually disappears.

The last secret, strontium and boron, will further harden the bones, and I would recommend that you add these too to get as much benefit as possible. Finally, I advise my patients not to take calcium carbonate (like Tums for the osteoporosis) because only 20 percent of it is absorbed. You can, however, use any other calcium salt, like calcium sulfate.

Sixteen

THE SECRETS OF THE ENDOCRINE SYSTEM

A hormone is defined as a chemical secreted by cells of one organ system that is released into the blood to be transported to another organ system where it will hook onto a receptor and then do whatever its chemistry is destined for. This scenario, which is played out all over the body, every minute of the day, is called the endocrine system. Here are some of its secrets.

Hormones really represent only a small share of nutritional therapies, but you would think otherwise because there are so many ads both on TV and the Internet for them. These are mostly bogus claims. You cannot take hormones orally, most of the time, because they are proteins and will become denatured when stomach acid destroys them. So forget about that oral testosterone supplement (too bad, guys, it's not that easy).

Before we go on to specific endocrine problems, let's take a look at the glands themselves. The pituitary gland is located in the brain behind the eyes. Anatomically, the crossover fibers from the retinal nerve sit in front of it, which is why any tumors of the pituitary cause lateral vision defects.

The pituitary, despite its small size, is an important gland because it releases stimulating hormones that signal other endocrine glands to release their hormones for the body to act on. It's on a negative feedback system, so when these other glands release their hormones, these hormones go back to the pituitary and turn the pituitary off. For example, the stimulating hormone for the thyroid is (TSH), adrenal cortical stimulating hormone is (ACTH) for cortisol and the luteinizing hormone (LH) for progesterone in the ovaries.

Finally, the pineal gland plays a role with melatonin for sleep. If melatonin is not released normally, this can increase cancer rates. Which will be discussed later.

Low Blood Pressure

Pathological low blood pressure is defined as a blood pressure less than 100 mmHg systolic (which is normally 120) and is associated with symptoms like dizziness and vertigo. It may be referred to as orthostatic, in that when you get up, your blood pressure will decrease further and lead to the symptoms. Patients, however, may have a systolic blood pressure of less than 100 mmHg, with no symptoms, which is normal. Therefore, the symptoms are key.

Medically, it's imperative that other causes of low blood pressure and dizziness (vertigo) are ruled out, like hypovolemia (decreased blood volume), high blood pressure medications, dehydration, bleeding, or anemia. That means that a thorough history and physical exam have to be done to rule out these and other medical conditions. Incidentally, Addison's disease, or a hypo- (low-) functioning adrenal gland with low cortisol levels, needs to be ruled out too, since it can cause a low blood pressure. President Kennedy had this condition and needed cortisone therapy to survive.

The secret here is that in the 1960s, a Russian scientist by the name of Vladimir Dilman wrote a paper called "The Health Project." In it, he concluded that aging was related to a drop-off of our hormones, in particular DHEA. DHEA stands for dihydroepiandrosterone, a hormone made in our adrenal gland that is a precursor for another 160 hormones, so it is very important and considered a progenitor. Low levels have been linked to lupus along with aging, low blood pressure states, and low testosterone levels. The DHEA can be easily measured as a standard blood test and as part of our general medical care. If blood levels of DHEA are low, replace it.

Another secret: don't buy the cheaper brands of DHEA, since many times they will not work in humans (only in rats) because we, as humans, don't have that rat enzyme to convert it. You will find these bogus preparations mostly in volume discount stores. The best, in my opinion, are the sublingual sprays (under the tongue).

Low-T syndrome can be helped, but first make sure that testosterone levels are low. As an aside, make sure that if you are testing for testosterone, you also check for estrogen, because if you are a man over forty, estrogen has to be lowered, and it can be done very nicely by taking Arimidex, an estrogen-blocking drug. It turns out that in some men, testosterone levels are low in the blood because testosterone is being siphoned off to make estrogen.

Pregnenolone, an adrenal hormone, is important in its relationship to stress reactions and maintenance of our cardiovascular system, including blood pressure. But the secret with its use is mostly related to a low blood pressure and muscle-wasting condition (sarcopenia). If patients develop a catabolic state in which they are losing weight and muscle mass, the pregnenolone can be of great value.

Finally, in patients with low blood pressures who are symptomatic, pregnenolone can raise the blood pressure and abort the symptoms associated with it. There is a medical condition called Shy-Drager syndrome in older patients with dizziness and low blood pressure where pregnenolone works nicely. In this scenario, many times I will use pregnenolone in tandem with branched-chain amino acids and DHEA. Lastly, in low-T or testosterone syndrome, I will use it with DHEA.

Growth hormone (GH), also called insulin growth factor, or IGF (which is its active ingredient), affects blood pressure too along with many other things. It's normally made in our brain, the pituitary, and secreted mostly at night. GH definitely decreases with age; binds to all tissues including the brain; and builds bones, muscles, and nerves. It also increases T-cell immunity and helps reduce cholesterol and LDL levels. Also, exercise performance improves, brain function gets better with increased focus and concentration, and breathing gets stronger.

The secret here is that blood levels need to be checked for GH, and, if low, replacement is necessary. Don't fall prey to these clinics, however, that proclaim longevity with intravenous replacement of growth hormone because they are expensive and dangerous. It's simple: have your doctor check your blood level, and if low with no contraindications, replace the GH sublingually (medication is placed under your tongue).

As an addendum, there may be some benefit with IGF for chronic fatigue, general medical care, Lou Gehrig's disease, and depression, where the growth hormone creates a wake-up-like state. They call this the Lazarus effect, described by Frank Herbert in his book *Dune*. Do you remember the movie?

In regard to aging and general medical care, I think growth hormone is a must, along with DHEA, lipoic acid, branched-chain amino acids, and other things that support the DNA, such as vitamin B3, vitamin B12, and folic acid. That means that with low blood levels of GH and no other medical problems present, GH should be replaced.

GH is a very important part of our physiology, but it's being abused too much by athletes who want to be better athletes, and by workout nutcases who want to body-beautify like me—but mine is natural! The end result is that these groups with their distorted minds make it bad for the people who can use GH and need it. It's like narcotics. The abusers have created an environment in which politicians, with their knee-jerk reflexes, have passed such strict laws that the patients who need the nutrients can't get them without sacrificing an arm and a leg, along with their doctors.

Why do you think we have pain centers all over the place making a gazillion dollars? Talk about medical costs going out of control! Now we have anesthesiologists charging hundreds to thousands of dollars for office visits and nerve blocks, when a visit with the primary-care doctor would have done it. By the way, recent studies reported that only 30 percent of patients with nerve blocks for back problems benefit. That means that 70 percent are a waste of health-care dollars, and 70 percent of patients are not getting better or finding relief for pain with their back problems.

Seventeen

THE SECRETS OF THE URINARY TRACT

The urinary tract is made up of the kidneys, ureters, urinary bladder, and the urethra (or tube that directs urine out of the body). I will stress the kidneys and bladder because they are the ones most affected and are very compliant to nutrients.

The major urinary tract problems that lend themselves to nutritional therapies are stone- and bladder-infection problems. Kidney stones are relatively common, with the most common being calcium oxalate. Triple phosphate and uric acid stones do occur, but they are rare and are generally seen in the context of repeated urinary infections or gout, respectively.

The secret with calcium oxalate stones is that the culprit is not the calcium, but the oxalate, so telling patients to stay away from calcium is not the answer. Instead, I advise them to *take* calcium, like Tums, with meals. Now why would I recommend that? The reason is that the calcium binds the oxalate in the food and makes it insoluble in the gastrointestinal tract, where it cannot be absorbed. When oxalate levels decrease in the bloodstream, the concentration of oxalate in the urine will also decrease, causing the stones to dissolve.

We have known for years that milk drinkers have fewer kidney stones, and this is the reason why. Calcium in the milk does that very thing. Many doctors still believe that calcium is the problem, but it isn't and does just the opposite.

By limiting calcium, the kidney-stone problem becomes worse. You, of course, need to drink a lot of water to keep the urine dilute, but the oxalate concentration is key. As an addendum, tea contains a lot of oxalate, whether it is hot or cold, so decrease its consumption.

The last secret is to make sure you do not have a parathyroid problem that can cause the kidney stones by elevating calcium levels. So a blood parathormone level is necessary to be sure. In addition, you can add two more secrets to the kidney-stone treatment with probiotics and cranberry extract, which help fight the infections that may occur and generally, at one time or another, are associated with stones.

Urinary Tract Infections (UTI)

The most common UTIs are bladder infections, but infections of the kidney do occur (pyelonephritis). They are much rarer, thank God, because they are much harder to treat. There is a linkage, however, because an untreated bladder infection can ascend up to the kidney via the ureter that drains the kidney, which means that all bladder infections need to be treated with vigor to avoid them.

The symptoms include increased urinating frequency, dysuria (burning during urination), fever, chills, and perhaps hematuria (or blood in the urine). A urine culture and sensitivity needs to be done and appropriate antibiotics taken. If the infection gets into the kidney, the ante goes up, and symptoms are much worse. Higher fever, chills, and back pain, which is in the midback area, not lower back, are its added symptoms, and they require IV antibiotics and a hospitalization.

The secret here is in using cranberry extract for the treatment *and* probiotics for the prevention of the problem. The cranberry extract, however, needs to be taken every twelve hours, because if you don't do so, the bacteria will gain access into the bladder wall and cause the infection. The cranberry works, but preventing the bacteria from adhering to the bladder wall thus prevents the colonization and infection of the bladder itself. The probiotic, two a day, on the other hand, can be taken either two at a time or better spread the capsules out (one twice a day).

Another secret is that cranberry extract (by the same mechanism) prevents H. pylori in the stomach from gaining access to the stomach wall and thereby prevents ulceration. Patients with recurrent UTIs or gastric/duodenal ulcers are told to take the cranberry indefinably for years, if necessary.

One more thing: the most common reason for women to have recurrent UTIs is poor hygiene. When cleaning themselves, they must be advised to wipe from front to back with only one swipe, and for each additional swipe, a new tissue is necessary. Auto-contamination is just common sense, but you would be surprised how many times this is the real problem, even with professionals such as female nurses.

In the long term, if you do not correct the problem, the chronic inflammation will predispose you to bladder stones and cancer of the bladder and kidneys. There's that chronic inflammation again! In this setting, the anti-inflammatory nutrients—such as resveratrol, curcumin, EPA, andrographia, and others—could be added.

Eighteen

THE SECRETS OF ALLERGIES

*O*ur immune systems protect us from outside invaders. Without this system, we could not survive. But when an outside invader becomes excessive, then we have problems that manifest as allergies. Even worse, over time, allergies can cause organ dysfunction and even cancer because of the ongoing inflammation.

Allergy

Allergy is an immune reaction of the body to any foreign agent that can manifest itself through many organ systems, such as the skin, throat, lungs, joints, gastro-intestinal tract, liver, and kidneys. Generally, when a foreign agent enters our bodies, it is taken up by our macrophages/dendritic cells and processed, so the body knows how to get rid of it. Either the T cells or the B cells that make anti-bodies are summoned to do the dirty work, but mast and basophile cells are also recruited, and these reactions cause the allergic (asthma) symptoms by releasing histamine. If IgA antibodies are recruited, then gastrointestinal symptoms arise, like abdominal pain and diarrhea.

Knowing this, the secret of treating allergies is to first identify them, then avoid them (which does not require a Rhodes Scholar to figure out), and then treat them as necessary. Remember, the body never forgets what is called the anamnestic response, and that is why bee stings or drug reactions are so danger-ous—because with every succeeding event, the body's reaction will be worse, even if it is years later.

Treatment medically will depend on what organ system is being affected and how severe the reaction is, but there are basic treatments that we can all use. Antihistamines, steroids, and other anti-inflammatory medications like an-tileukotriens (Singulair, a drug for asthma, for example) are used medically, but nutritionally, there are other secret remedies.

Quercetin, found in apples and onions, is a powerful anti-allergy agent that is very useful in preventing and treating allergies. It reduces the intensity of the symptoms along with decreasing the incidence of attacks. Resveratrol along with curcumin may have some benefit since they both inhibit NFkB (nuclear factor kappa beta), a powerful chemical in the play-out of inflammation—that word again, *inflammation*. Finally, butterbur, synergistically along with quercetin, is useful for prevention and treatment, with butterbur also being effective for migraine.

The bottom line is when you hear the word *allergy*, think nutrients that universally can be used to prevent and treat all of them, regardless of the organ system affected. Just as an aside, one of the most common allergies that I see is to mold, mildew, and mites. The mold and mildew can occur anywhere, but here in Florida, it is a given with our tropical weather.

Mites are microscopic, spider-looking creatures that live in our beds and eat the skin cells that we desquamate (scale off) when we are sleeping. You can't see mites, but they hook onto dust particles (dust mites) and float around while you are sleeping, and you breathe them in. When this happens, you react to them with typically allergic symptoms in the morning when you get up.

Mold, mildew, and mites can be diagnosed with blood tests and, if posi-tive, avoided. If the funguses (mold and mildew) are positive, change your air-conditioning filters every month and have your ducts checked for them. If the mites are positive, you need to vacuum your bed three times a week and put a HEPA filter near your side of the bed and run it twenty-four hours a day. That will take out particles and dust where the mites are riding. If you go to Walmart or Costco, you can get a HEPA filter at reasonable prices. If that doesn't work, you can get a humidistat and put it on your air-conditioning thermostats for your bedroom and set it at less than 40 percent. Mites cannot live with humidity of less than 40 percent, so if your bedroom is less than that, they will die, and your allergies will go away. Lastly, for seasonal allergies, quercetin, vitamin C (2,000 mg once a day for women or 3,000 mg once a day for men), and butterbur are my choices. For bee strings, which can be fatal, keep your EpiPen handy!

Nineteen

The reason why this chapter title is so exaggerated is that each area represents a small part of nutrient treatments, and if I separated them, there would be ten more chapters. Also, they have some shared benefits, so it's a better fit.

Headaches

Headaches are a common complaint, and the secrets with them include establishing a diagnosis and knowing what nutrients will help. The most common headaches are secondary to stress and sinus-related problems. Once the primary or root cause is found, it needs to be treated, and the headache will go away. Don't forget that hypertension will also cause headaches, along with brain tumors, so please get your blood pressure checked. The last severe headache patient I had was being treated for migraines, and when the hypertension was treated, the headaches went away. The secret is to treat the root cause.

Migraines

Migraines have a typical presentation in that they generally involve one side of the brain and may have an aura (a sensation that a headache is on the way, as a warning), and the patients have nausea with photophobia (light hurts their eyes). Generally, because the symptoms are so severe, a brain scan (MRI) is done to rule out a brain tumor. Treatment is begun with a standard regimen of triptans (Maxalt), beta-blockers (Atenolol), and nonsteroidal analgesics (Motrin).

The gigantic secret here is that nutritional therapy is generally as good as the standard, expensive medication and produces no side effects. Feverfew and butterbur are well tolerated, cheap, and essentially side-effect-free. At the last meeting I went to regarding migraine headaches, the medical headache expert agreed that the butterbur was very effective and perhaps just as effective as the standard medications that he was lecturing on. Hurrah for the good guys!

An additional secret with migraines is that the treatment has to be started *early*, and not after the migraine has set in. Also, when buying butterbur, read the label and make sure that it is pyrrolizidine-free, which can be toxic. Finally, if you are a woman on estrogen (birth control pills) and having migraines, they should be discontinued because birth control pills are a risk factor for a stroke.

Sinus Headaches

The sinuses are located over the frontal skull areas (over the eyes) and under our eyes, which are the maxillary sinuses. These headaches typically are throbbing and are made worse with lying down and smoking. The pain is exacerbated by gently percussing (tapping over the painful area with a finger) on exam. Secondary to bacteria, fungus, smoking, and allergy, steroids and antibiotics are used along with nasal steroid aerosol-inhalation treatments. From a nutritional standpoint, anti-inflammatories like quercetin, curcumin, and resveratrol may help even prevent the problem. Studies have not been done yet, but these nutrients make sense.

Tension Headaches

Tension headaches are common and characteristically occur later in the day when the stress is most profound. They are located over the back of the neck area. Such a headache feels "spastic," and that is exactly what it is. The stress, either mental or physical, leads to muscle spasm, which causes the pain. By the way, computers have made tension headaches even worse because of users' poor posture and inappropriate screen alignment. Passion flower and ashwagandha are the nutritional secrets that will help relieve the spasm and tension and thereby prevent and decrease the headaches. Lavender and lemon balms are also relaxing and helpful.

High Blood Pressure Headaches

These headaches tend to be global, or all over the head, and are directly linked to the degree of blood pressure elevation (in other words, lower the pressure, and the headache will improve). They tend to be throbbing and at times associated with visual symptoms like blurring. With the standard blood pressure medications, CoQ10, PQQ, taurine, and hawthorn can be useful adjuncts or can be used by themselves if the blood pressure is not too high.

The worst-case scenario would be to get an erroneous normal blood pressure recording from an automated blood pressure machine at the grocery or drugstore, where you put your arm into this device, and then not get treated for the high blood pressure that you really have. That is a prescription for disaster—a preventable one.

I am going to digress a moment to go over hypertension more thoroughly. There are two types of hypertension. The first is "essential." We do not know the cause of this type, but it accounts for up to 95 percent of people with high blood pressure. The second is "nonessential," which makes up 5 percent of people where there is a known cause, such as adrenal gland problems.

Regardless, most times there are no symptoms, so a physical exam would be necessary to diagnose it. Your doctor's job is to diagnose your high blood pressure, separate essential from nonessential, and then treat it. If you have symptoms, they would include headaches, dizziness, bloody nose, and shortness of breath, but without treatment, heart disease, strokes, and kidney failure with early death are its legacy.

Lungs

I have already discussed lung cancer, which leaves everything else, and almost everything else that causes diseases of the lungs is either indirectly or directly related to inflammation. That word again! The lungs function to exchange O_2 with CO_2, but you must remember that the lungs and heart are interconnected through the blood supply, so anything that affects one will affect the other.

For example, in congestive heart failure, blood will start reversing, or backing up into the lungs, and will lead to fluid accumulation and shortness of breath. Here the lungs are not the problem, so our remedy would be to treat the heart disease first. In addition, the lungs have an immense environmental exposure, so with every breath we take, allergy and environmental concerns are important considerations.

The secret with lung disease is inflammation, whether it is acute or chronic, so our natural remedies can play a significant role. More recently, even the medical profession itself has introduced Daliresp, a drug that works by reducing inflammation as its sole mode of action. Can you imagine that! The most common diseases are bacterial or viral infections, so appropriate antibiotics and antivirals are the treatment of choice.

Also, in chronic fatigue syndrome, which can cause repeated lung infections, nutrients should play a major role in both treatment and prevention. Resveratrol, curcumin (anti N.F.k.B. agents), ginseng, fucoidans, reishi/cistanche, and branched-chain amino acids with high doses of vitamin C (3,000–5,000mg/day) would be recommended. Two herpes viruses, Epstein-Barr and cytomegalic, are responsible, and the nutrients decrease their replication. Here you can see that both conditions need to be treated: the organism and the target organ (the lungs).

For people with chronic and long-standing inflammatory problems like emphysema, COPD (chronic obstructive lung disease), asthma, sarcoid, and bronchiectasis, this regimen is good and only makes sense with the addition of glutathione, cysteine, and EPA. The secret with the glutathione and cysteine is that they are long-term antioxidants that target our lungs. The body makes these nutrients (in the liver) but in this case becomes overwhelmed by free radicals and needs to be supplemented.

In summary, the goal again is to treat the inflammation aggressively, so as to prevent chronic inflammation that can lead to scarring, lung dysfunction, and even cancer of the lung. We as physicians treat these chronic lung conditions with long-term steroids as anti-inflammatory agents that have immense consequences when we could be using natural, less dangerous modalities like these nutrients.

Asthma

Asthma is also a chronic inflammatory condition of the lung, but due to allergy. As a result of the allergen-allergic reaction, inflammatory proinflammates (chemicals) are released that cause the asthmatic symptoms (such as shortness of breath, wheezing requiring steroids, inhalers, and antibiotics) over and over again.

There are two types of asthma: intrinsic, where no allergen can be found; and extrinsic, where an allergen can be identified and treatment would include trying to find out what you are allergic to, in order to avoid it. The secret is that these proinflammates, or inflammatory chemicals, like tumor necrosis factor (TNF) and interleukin, can be treated with curcumin, mung bean, resveratrol, cysteine, and glutathione to prevent or ameliorate the symptoms, requiring less medication and avoiding the chronic long-term consequences like emphysema and COPD.

Again, in summary, with asthma, treat the root problem, which is an allergic proinflammatory etiology (cause), and avoid the long-term consequences.

Premenstrual and Postmenopausal Syndromes

I grouped two maladies together (PMS and menopause) because they have many similarities and are easily explained together.

PMS, or premenstrual syndrome, occurs in premenstrual women who have irritability, abdominal pain, headaches, and many other related symptoms just prior to the start of their menstrual period. It is believed that the hormone shifts are the reason why, but it is not well understood.

Standard medical therapy with tranquilizers and nonsteroidal analgesics is used, but many times such treatment is ineffective, and the patient is dismissed and considered nonfunctional. The secret here is that, depending on how severe the symptoms are, I generally begin with flax seed and follow it with black cohosh, soy, and green tea. Flax seed has several "good guys" in it, with phytoestrogens or lignans being relevant here. The most active ingredient is alpha linoleic acid (ALA), an omega-6 oil that's converted to an omega-3 oil and that is anti-inflammatory.

The Mayo Clinic did a study using flax seed and found that five tablespoons a day decreased PMS symptoms by 60 percent. The flax seed has to be chewed or ground, however, prior to consumption to release the phytoestrogens and lignans that fill the estrogen receptors to alleviate the symptoms. In addition, the alpha linoleic acid in it converts to the omega-3 oils and, therefore, is very anti-inflammatory, which may also help. The problem is that only 20 percent is converted to the omega-3 oils, and the remaining 80 percent is of no use.

Black cohosh, or cimicifuga racemose, can also be a useful adjunct by stabilizing luteinizing hormone (LH) and estrogen levels, and the active ingredient is vitexin. It has been my experience that black cohosh is very well tolerated, cheap, and without side effects.

Finally, soy and green tea, which again go back to Southeast Asia, where women there experience very few of the PMS and menopausal symptoms, decrease the estrogen effects by filling up the estrogen receptors and blocking them while maintaining the ratio of estrone (weak estrogen) to estradiol (strong estrogen). Soy's active ingredients (phytoestrogens) are genistin, daidzein, and equol, while in green tea, EGCG (epigallocatechin gallate), a polyphenol, helps correct the hormonal imbalance along with an anti-inflammatory action.

The secret here is that this regimen works, is cheap, poses little risk, and can be used in tandem to treat symptoms. Unfortunately for women, many doctors dismiss these symptoms, and as a result, women are told to live with them. One last thing: this regimen may decrease the effectiveness of birth control pills, so be careful and practice protected sex.

As stated earlier, menopause has many similarities to PMS, but the physiology is completely different. Here women experience hot flashes, fatigue, irritability, and muscle aches and pains because of low estrogen levels, and when estrogen is replaced, symptoms improve. There is a great deal of controversy regarding estrogen replacement, but as of today, low-dose estrogen replacement for less than ten years is not a risk for breast cancer.

If the uterus is intact, then progesterone will also be necessary; otherwise, you will start to have your periods. The secret here is that a nutritional supplement with flax seed, soy, and green tea would be a better choice along with the benefit of preventing breast cancer. Just ask those women in Southeast Asia. The soy and green tea act like estrogens, fill those same receptors, and thereby decrease menopause symptoms, with no risk. It's safe and cheap—not bad!

Sleep

Sleep is a normal part of our physiology and is required to replace cellular fatigue proteins and excrete the waste products of our metabolic engines. Studies have been done on keeping people awake, and guess what? After two to three days, they cannot stay awake. Some of the things already discussed in this chapter, such as headaches, sinus headaches, menopause, PMS, and asthma, may interfere with sleep and must be dealt with if sleep is to improve.

Normal sleep requires that we go through phases, with at least two of them being REM (rapid eye movement) sleep. This phase is where we dream, and if people do not dream, then they may be lacking in this component and not getting enough sleep. When we go to sleep and it is dark out, our body releases melatonin from the pineal gland in the brain, which helps with the sleep process. If melatonin is not released on a daily basis, there are other surprising implications.

Night workers who do not release melatonin, for example, have a 30 percent increased risk of developing cancers of the colon, lung, and pancreas. It's believed that melatonin has an anticancer effect, which leads us to the supposition that lack of it in these types of scenarios would require replacement, and I would agree.

In dealing with sleep-related problems, a thorough medical history is required. We need to know if patients are taking any stimulants (caffeine); working out in the evening; taking too many naps, especially in the afternoon; not sleeping in a sleep-inducing room (dark, no lights, with the radio, TV, e-book devices, and computers off); or taking other medications that may interrupt sleep. By the way, electronic books give off a blue light that disrupts melatonin release, so don't use them either.

Doctors will want to know if you snore, indicating possible sleep apnea. Sleeping medications should not be used every night (every other night is OK), because they are addicting. If taken every night, they will become ineffective (tachyphylaxis), and you will have to take more. The secret here is a nutritional supplement such as melatonin, which will work great or not at all (my experience). There is no in-between. Also, valerian, passion flower, lemon balm, and lavender are useful adjuncts and can be used in combination. One word of advice: the valerian stinks, so don't smell the bottle. Galen called it "phu," (bad odor) and for good reason.

Anxiety and Depression

These two problems are not only common, but many times are expressed in the same person. Knowing that, it is important clinically that they be separated and treated as separate entities, because if you don't, it will become very confusing, and the treatment will not be satisfactory.

Anxiety is a hyperkinetic state both mentally and physically in which the patient becomes worried, with some loss of control about things in his or her life that are for the most part commonplace. If anxiety becomes severe enough, the patient will become nonfunctional, and a depression may follow.

Therefore, the secret is to treat the anxiety effectively so that the depression will not occur. If they do coexist, then they both need to be treated. Standard anxiety medication works (drugs such as Xanax, Valium, and Ativan), but patients can become dependent and even addicted to them if the patients are not careful.

A deep secret is that anxiety can be treated nutritionally, without the worry of addiction or side effects that may affect people's jobs or driving, because these nutrients do not cloud mental function or impair reflex time. As mentioned, ashwagandha and passion flower are the two nutritional supplements that I recommend, along with a historical review of what is making a patient anxious. It's important because in doing so and by identifying triggers, the patient is more likely to deal with them by avoiding or solving the problem, and then the anxiety will go away or improve.

The same is true for depression. By sorting out the reasons why someone is depressed, you can then correct the problem without or with less medicine that would be ordinarily necessary. Also, depression occurs because of a hormonal imbalance in the brain among serotonin, epinephrine, and dopamine—all neurotransmitters (brain wave activity).

Nutritionally, with depression, St. John's Wort and SAMe (s-adenosylmethionine) are very effective. They are best used early, however, in the course of depression, because they will be more effective, with the only caveat being that SAMe is expensive. It's interesting because SAMe physiologically works exactly the same as the standard medications such as Lexapro, Effexor, and Zoloft by inhibiting serotonin uptake in the brain. SAMe can be used as an add-on to the standard medications.

A secret note of interest: St. John's Wort is called that because it comes from a flower that blooms only on St. John's birthday (June 24) and from *wort*, which is Old English for *plant*. Because of many drug interactions with St. John's Wort, I do not recommend it to anyone taking any other medication.

Nails and Hair

Now, why would I group nails with hair? The reason is that both are scleroproteins and, as a result, respond the same way to therapy. The thinning of our fingernails or brittle nails and the thinning of our hair, which is called alopecia, is secondary to different reasons, but the end result is the same.

The secret here is that grape-seed extract works for both hair and nails, but it may take two to three months to work, so be patient. In contrast, alopecia can be due to many things, like chemicals that they use with our hair products such as dyes, rinses, and conditioners, along with stress, which are the most common reasons for hair loss. Lupus erythematosus, an autoimmune disease, also causes hair loss, so the disease must be ruled out, especially in women. With lupus and the other autoimmune disease too, peony extract, mung bean extract, and DHEA (dehydroepiandrosterone) might help. In men, on the other hand, a hereditary problem carried in the mother's lineage is the main reason why they become bald. Here the hair nerve roots are being destroyed by testosterone, so Propecia is the drug of choice, which blocks the testosterone effect.

The secret here in men is that saw palmetto will block the testosterone in a similar way, which will improve the alopecia. Again, since hair grows so slowly, you'll need to wait two to three months to see an effect. As an added benefit, saw palmetto will shrink the prostate through the same mechanism of testosterone blockage that we use on men with benign prostatic enlargement (BPH).

Finally, with skin bleeding and capillary fragility that causes bruising in older people or people on aspirin, grape-seed extract will reverse bleeding. In addition, if taking aspirin, which can do it also, a decrease in dose to every three to four days may also help yet maintain the aspirin benefit. In this way, important drugs like aspirin don't have to be stopped, thus endangering the patient. Finally, as an addendum for skin bleeding and capillary fragility, vitamin C (2,000 mg per day for women and 3,000 mg per day for men) will help.

General Medical Care

This is probably the most important category because it pertains to everyone, even if you are feeling well, whether you are young or old, male or female. General care is related to aging, so a review of aging itself, along with antioxidants and free radicals, needs be explained. Therefore, I want you to pay attention!

Aging is now a relevant topic and not just a fait accompli, so understanding it will make my recommendations more understandable and relevant. We now know that our organ systems (brain, heart, lungs, and kidneys, for example) will replace themselves through their own cellular DNA, as long as they have the raw materials for their metabolic engines or if they become diseased. It goes without saying that avoiding diseases that could damage these same cells promotes the value of that yearly history and physical exam. For example, on average, our kidneys and liver will replace themselves every eight years, and our hearts every twenty-eight years. Don't forget to exercise (both aerobic, weight resistance, and yoga for stretching and balance) and follow a proper diet to help maintain blood flow to these organs.

One mechanism that affects our cellular DNA and stops it from functioning normally is telomeres, or the ends of our DNA strands that become shortened as we get older. When shortened, the same DNA in our cells cannot replace themselves as quickly, so the cells become dysfunctional and start to die. Electronic magnetic fields in computers, TVs, routers, Wi-Fi, and cell phones, along with free radicals, alcohol, smoking, chemicals, and many other things shorten those telomeres. Nutrients can be very useful here by up-regulating the good genes and down-regulating the bad genes to avoid the shortening. Nutrients would include resveratrol, PQQ, CoQ10, pterostilbene, folic acid, and B12.

Another reason for aging is the loss of our mitochondria. Mitochondria are tiny organelles in every cell (between two to two thousand five hundred in each cell), which have their own DNA (they do not share the cells' nuclear DNA). So what does that tell you? It tells you that our "Maker" paid special attention to them, because they make the energy so that the cell can do what it does and also reproduce itself. It's like the gas tanks in our cars, because if you run out of gas, the car will not run, and neither will your cells if these energy producers are not protected. They do it by making a chemical ATP (adenosine Tri-phosphate). But the mitochondria start to disappear with the aging process for the same reasons that affect our telomeres.

We now know, however, that these mitochondria can be protected and also will increase in number with nutritional supplements, in a process that is called biogenesis, which has created a whole new field of study. The secret here is that lipoic acid, branched-chain amino acid, acetylcholine, CoQ10, and PQQ will do this very thing in the realm of biogenics, and the hope is to protect the mitochondria we have and produce more. The more gas we have, the farther the car will go!

The third mechanism that I have already alluded to is the decline of our hormones as we age. As mentioned earlier, Dr. Vladimir Dilman in the 1960s was the first to note hormone drop-offs with age—and more specifically loss of DHEA. This has been established for other hormone systems too, and we need to check for them with blood analysis and, if low, replace them. DHEA, testosterone, estrogen, growth hormone, cortisol, and thyroid are just a few and can contribute greatly to the aging process. Make this part of your yearly exam and "plug the holes" of your endocrine dysfunction.

The last important reason for aging is disease. How many times have you heard, "Look how much he has aged after that heart attack!" Human diseases in and by themselves will age you because of the oxidative stress damage that your cellular systems encounter, but as an extension of this premise, can antioxidants in your body protect you and prevent any oxidative process that might affect you in the future?

Dr. Frank Wilczek, a professor of physics at MIT, might serve as a good example and help us with at least a cocktail that he takes to ward off aging and this oxidative process. He won the Nobel Prize in physics at the age of twenty-three while a graduate student at Princeton when he discovered quarks and their influence on neutrons and protons. Therefore, he should be smart enough to know what to take. Specifically, he takes vitamin B12, folic acid, K2, acetylcarnitine, lipoic acid, EPA, and vitamin C.

I would respectively agree and disagree with him because my recommendations would *also* include resveratrol with pterostilbene, curcumin, CoQ10, PQQ, pomegranate, branched-chain amino acids, and bilberry. This secret recommendation is for a healthy person, so if that same person has other medical problems, of course, there would be add-ons. I know that it sounds like a lot, but if you develop what I call "the grazing technique" and spread them out throughout the day, it's not too burdensome and will make a great difference over time.

This secret, magic cocktail will provide the essential nutrients that your body needs for those metabolic engines, protect your telomeres, maintain and make new mitochondria (through biogenesis), and neutralize any free radicals that might be floating around and causing cellular damage.

Twenty

The Secrets of the Gastrointestinal Tract (GI Tract)

I am a gastroenterologist, so this subject is near and dear to me. I am also an internist, which is the study of the esophagus, stomach, small intestine, large intestine, liver, and pancreas. Nutrients are making great strides recently in regard to preventing and treating all kinds of diseases that I will review here.

Gastrointestinal Disorders

I have already discussed cancers of the GI tract, but there is much more to discuss. The anatomical geography will lend to your understanding of GI disorders, so let's start from the top and work down, clockwise from left to right.

The most frequent complaint of GI disorders is abdominal pain. Before we begin, let me review a Duke University study that was reported twenty years ago that concluded that *where* the abdominal pain was coming from was the best way to make a correct diagnosis. That means that finding the location will lead you and me alike to the root cause and appropriate treatment. Believe it or not, pain is better than any x-rays, lab tests, other physical findings or history offered.

That reminds me of another secret. It is essential that we treat the root cause of any problem and not the symptoms, which is a mistake made by many physicians. So make sure your doctor is always a "root cause" kind of person.

Upper-Abdominal Pain

Upper-abdominal pain, or epigastric pain, is generally caused by an underlying gastric (stomach), pancreas, duodenal, or esophageal problem. The secret in differentiating them is associated symptoms. For example, with esophageal problems, there will also be problems with swallowing or dysphasia. Stomach ulcerations are made worse with eating; whereas duodenal ulcers are made better with food. Typically, duodenal ulcers wake people up during the night because that's when the acid levels in your duodenum are the highest.

After a standard work-up, which may include an upper endoscopy and biopsy, nutritional therapies may be of great use. For esophageal problems, curcumin, resveratrol, and green-tea supplements are anti-inflammatory and may help prevent cancer conversion that we see with Barrett's esophagus—a premalignant (leads to cancer) condition. For the gastric (stomach) or duodenal ulcers, green tea, olive oil, and deglycyrrhized licorice would be indicated.

Finally, cranberry extract here prevents the H. pylori bacteria from gaining access into the gastric mucosa, which can cause an ulcer, and therefore may be a useful adjunct since these bacteria have been related not only to gastric ulcers, but to cancer of the stomach. As mentioned, olive oil will do the same and is anti-inflammatory to boot, so it's a good add-on. Just drink one to two ounces three times a day with food, and it works, along with a thank-you from your cardiovascular system.

Pancreatitis, or inflammation of the pancreas, can also present as epigastric pain, nausea, and emesis (vomiting), but characteristically the pain radiates straight through into the back. The condition is related to increased alcohol consumption, elevated triglyceride levels, cancer of the pancreas, cytomegalic virus, elevated IgG levels (an antibody), and diabetes mellitus. It is not to be trifled with since people can die from pancreatitis, so a medical treatment needs to be seriously administered and followed.

Treatment secrets involve treating the underlying condition, along with pancreatic enzyme replacement and nutritional supplements, but the secret here is that the medications come first, before the nutritional supplements. Remember, pancreatitis can be fatal! Licorice and green tea may be useful adjuncts, in addition to stopping the alcohol and lowering the triglyceride levels, along with diet and medication.

The final secret is that cancer of the pancreas has been linked to chronic relapsing pancreatitis, so if the condition is recurrent, consider GLA (gamma linoleic acid), curcumin, and soy protein. As a corollary, I would recommend this nutritional regimen for any patient at risk for cancer of the pancreas, which I had outlined earlier as a preventive measure.

Upper-Left Quadrant

Upper-left-quadrant pain occurs infrequently, mainly because there is not much there, but when it becomes an issue, we need to think of an enlarged spleen or problems with the left colon. To sort out the nature of the problem, a CT scan of the abdomen and rarely a colonoscopy would be necessary, upon which therapy would be implemented.

One condition, however, that causes upper-left-quadrant pain can be managed with nutrients and diet alone, and it is called splenic flexure syndrome. These patients complain of gas-like pain with constipation. Most tests are negative, but abdominal x-rays will show a dilated colon under the left diaphragm that's causing the pain. A variant of irritable bowel syndrome, it is treated with fiber replacement along with probiotics to increase transit bowel times and decompress that left colon.

A more recent secret is adding peppermint extract to increase transit time and help ameliorate the symptoms. Fiber can also be increased in the form of a high-fiber diet and flax seed, which must be ground up or chewed when consumed. The secret is that, in general, the natural remedies are generally better here than the standard medicines that we prescribe. If it is a spleen problem with enlargement, then a more thorough work-up will be necessary with the involvement of a hematologist/oncologist.

Kidney stones on either the right or the left side may cause a severe colicky (comes and goes) pain in this area, with blood in the urine (may be microscopic). Pain may radiate into the back, lower quadrants, or groin areas. The secret is that a urine analysis for RBC (red blood cells), a kidney ultrasound and a CT scan would be diagnostic. Antibiotics, fluids, cranberry extract, and probiotics will then be necessary. Seeing an urologist is helpful.

To prevent kidney stones, consider chewing Tums with meals to bind with oxalate in the food and make it insoluble. The secret is that, in doing this, oxalate can't be absorbed (oxalate becomes insoluble), resulting in a drop of blood level, which will then help reabsorb the oxalate in the stones to dissolve them. That along with an increase in water consumption is a must. We have known for a long time that milk drinkers have a low incidence of kidney stones, and because the calcium in the milk absorbs the oxalate out of the food, Tums does the same thing. But we (the medical profession) told people not to drink milk because of the lipid-heart risks, which was wrong. As a result, we have created a whole new generation of patients with kidney stones.

Lower-Left Quadrant

Lower-left-quadrant pain is very common and therefore has significant implications. There are many etiologies or causes, so it is imperative that a good work-up be done, which would include blood tests, CT scans, and, if indicated, a colonoscopy. With an acute inflammatory process, a colonoscopy may actually be contraindicated until the inflammation decreases because of the risk of perforation of the colon.

From inflammatory colitis to diverticulitis, an assortment of diseases needs to be ruled out, but since it would be impossible to review all of them, the two most common are worth going over. Diverticula of the colon occur to a great extent in all of us as Americans because of our low-fiber diets that result in high-pressure areas of the left colon, causing outpouching. They look like mushrooms attached to the outside of a bowl. These herniations, or diverticula, can bleed, become infected, or potentially rupture. Urgent medical therapy may be needed to avoid possible surgery, which could include a colostomy (wearing a bag).

The secret here is that once the acute diverticular problem is completely treated medically with antibiotics, antispasmodics, and probiotics and when symptoms are gone, then flax seed, wheat grass, and phloridzin that release butyrate (decrease inflammation of the lining cells in the bowel), along with a high-fiber diet, can help prevent the next exacerbation. I agree with the old advice of staying away from nuts and popcorn, since I have seen exacerbation after ingestion, and of course it makes sense.

Since the long-term risk of this may be cancer of the colon, cruciferous extracts with beta-carotene, applewise polyphenol extracts containing suforaphanes, beta isothiocyanates, and apigenin would be also recommended. The secret is again prevention of the acute and long-term problems, including colon rupture and cancer, which can be dreadful.

If the left-lower-quadrant pain is due to inflammatory colitis, than ulcerative and Crohn's disease would be the most common diagnoses. The most common symptom besides the pain is bloody diarrhea. The standard medications would include steroids and nonabsorbable antibiotics and, if necessary, immune suppressants (decreases immunity), but the secret is that nutrients are a much-needed adjunct (help), and they work. Folic acid, probiotics, vitamin B12, and EPA (omega-3 oils) along with wheat grass will not only help decrease symptoms and relapses, but also will result in much less need for the standard medications, thereby decreasing unwanted side effects and costs.

Many times I have seen patients treated like this to remission (to become symptom-free) and be maintained on only the nutrients for long periods of time. Since the ulcerative-colitis variety may be related to colon cancer, prevention along with anti-inflammatory effects could be accomplished with curcumin, resveratrol, cruciferous vegetables or extract, and applewise phenolic extracts. More recently, I would add mung bean extract for its cytokine (inflammatory chemicals) "cooling effect." These extracts work through NFkB, which stands for nuclear factor kappa beta, a nuclear transcriptor enzyme that can convert the colon cell from an inflammatory one to a cancerous one by blocking it. In summary, the secrets lie with both short- and long-term nutrients.

Lower-Right Quadrant

Lower-right-abdominal pain includes everything I have discussed already in regard to irritable bowel syndrome, Crohn's disease, and ulcerative colitis, but now we need to add appendicitis. When I was a resident, they taught us that someone with lower-right-abdominal pain who lost his or her appetite had appendicitis until proven otherwise, and I have found that to be true. That's a big secret!

Appendicitis is diagnosed by CT scan, which is the diagnostic test of choice, and then it's treated with antibiotics and surgery as soon as possible. It can be a medical emergency if rupture occurs, so a prompt diagnosis is imperative. Another, more recent secret here has to do with a recent finding that the appendix is not just a vestigial (useless) organ or appendage, but a primary source of our own probiotics. That tells us that we need to preserve the appendix, if possible, and not take it out incidentally because we are surgically in the area.

For example, when a woman is undergoing gynecological surgery, the appendix will be removed very commonly just because the surgeon is in the area, in order to presumably prevent a future acute appendicitis. It's also important to know that vitamin B12 is absorbed in the terminal ileum, which is in the lower part of the small bowel just before the colon begins in the lower-right quadrant. Any problem here, like Crohn's disease, could cause a vitamin B12 deficiency. In that case, B12 needs to be replaced to avoid pernicious anemia.

Upper-Right Quadrant

Upper-right-quadrant pain is almost always related to the gallbladder. True, kidney stones and liver disease can also cause this pain, but the gallbladder needs to be our first concern. In medical school we were taught a mnemonic that goes like this: fertile, fat, forty, flatulent (gas) in a female generally describes how gallbladder disease presents with the pain of course in the URQ, which is a very common scenario. The pain may also radiate back into the right shoulder blade, along with nausea.

There generally is a strong family history of gallstones, especially with the mother or her side of the family. Gallstones, if symptomatic (pain, nausea, vomiting), must be surgically removed, which can be done laparoscopically, and only requires a one- to two-day hospitalization. If patients have asymptomatic gallstones, then generally we don't operate, and patients are watched carefully for any symptoms (and then gallstones must come out).

An important secret and exception: diabetics with gallstones and no symptoms have to have them removed because of the high complication rate if they wait. That's the art of medicine and knowing disease processes.

Nutritionally, the secrets here are lipotain (tree-gum guggal extract) and red-yeast rice, which will decrease cholesterol in the blood and also in the gallbladder that may, in fact, prevent or shrink the stones, since most stones are cholesterol-based. Certain medications, like bile salts or statins taken orally, will also help wash out or prevent the formation of cholesterol that makes the stones. For the chronic inflammation, I would recommend curcumin, resveratrol, PQQ, mung bean extract, and quercetin because the chronic inflammatory component is also linked to cancer of the gallbladder. Here again, the secret of treating today's simple problem is to prevent tomorrow's tragic, more complicated, expensive, and potentially deadly problem. Axiom: "To prevent is better than to treat."

Now that you have gone around the horn in regard to gastrointestinal disease, you can see how location of the pain is the secret to the diagnosis, which will lead you and your physician to the correct treatment and nutrients to use. Obviously, it is the doctor's responsibility to make the correct diagnosis, but sometimes he or she will need some help! Since you are on the receiving end of this medical care, I think that the secrets discussed here may potentially make your care better and allow you to live longer and healthier. Your history that the doctor asks for will now be more informative and be more relevant. Like a successful Hilton Hotel parallel, think location, location, location when it comes to gastrointestinal disease, and you will more likely to diagnose what's wrong.

Twenty-One

The Secrets of the Skin

If I asked you what the largest organ of our body is, you probably would have guessed the liver. Yes, the liver is very large, but the skin is the correct answer. It's much more than just a covering and is a one-way secreting membrane, like a Donnan membrane that we use in chemistry class.

Through sweating, the skin functions as an excreter of substances, like our kidneys do, that may be harmful to the body and also helps with thermal (temperature) control. Our core temperature is important because all of our body chemistries are based on it. Any fluctuation up or down will influence them and can lead to organ dysfunction or disease. Also, in our perspiration, water and electrolytes are removed from our bodies, thus decreasing our core temperature and preventing overheating. When you get a chance, just taste your sweat, and you will realize how salty (sodium) it is.

Our skin, however, will also age like all other organ systems unless we protect it from chemicals, free radicals, and the radiation effects of the sun. Yes, put suntan lotion with a high SPF (greater than 40, with zinc in it) on when at the beach, every two hours or after coming out of the water. Linked to this, of course, is the dreaded melanoma—a malignant skin cancer that deserves its reputation because it is highly invasive, metastasizes early, and can recur many years later (up to forty years).

The cells of our skin are no different than any other cell in our body, with their own DNA, replication, and renewal process, but direct exposure to the environment adds an important consideration. Skin cells also divide very slowly, so their metabolism is also slow, and response rates will take time and be delayed. Any harmful exposure on the skin can directly affect the skin and sometimes get absorbed into the bloodstream, with systemic effects. For example, volatile organic chemicals like acetone, formaldehyde, and solvents can affect our bone marrow or brain and have been directly liked to Parkinsonism.

I think we are all aware of avoiding excessive sun exposure, but the secret of nutrient therapy for the skin is about to be revealed. Grape-seed extract with its strong antioxidant activity has a predilection for the skin, and thus its beneficial effects include antiaging, promoting nail and hair growth, and preserving capillary fragility in the skin that prevents bleeding into the skin that we have discussed earlier—a condition that occurs as our skin ages.

Grape-seed extract may be a secret, until now, but the lycopene secret is even newer. We find lycopene principally in tomatoes. It is fat-soluble, so it has to be ingested with a fat-soluble agent like cheese (in pizza) and is found also in the skin of the tomato, which also protects it from the sun. Lycopene is released with cooking, so cooking tomatoes increases their benefit to you. Better cooked than raw.

Researchers at Mount Sinai Hospital in New York found that an enzyme in lycopene called ornithine decarboxylase, when applied directly to the skin, maintained its DNA and also stabilized the DNA's double-strand break-repair pathway. That means that the lycopene protection from the tomato and our skin's DNA results from activation of its own internal DNA pathway of repair. This same study also showed that the ultraviolet damage to the skin's DNA by depleting PCNA (proliferating-cell nuclear antigen) was reversed by applying the lycopene to the skin. It's a white, creamy extract that gets absorbed into the skin for its effect.

Therefore, lycopene, by improving cell-to-cell communication at gap junctions, decreases the harmful effects of oxidation on the skin. This helps with skin-cell growth and reproduction, along with down-regulating collagenase that destroys the skin's connective tissue, which results in wrinkles and aging of the skin. What this all means is that lycopene (found in red peppers and tomatoes, for example) is great for the skin in protecting it and allowing it to reproduce itself to stay healthy—meaning less cancer risk and wrinkles.

To summarize the secrets related to the largest organ of our body, think antioxidants, DNA, anti-inflammation, and protection. Lycopene, grape-seed extract, curcumin, resveratrol, quercetin, and andrographia would be a good approach, with the lycopene being rubbed on and also taken orally. The oral lycopene should be taken with supper since it is fat-soluble, like vitamin E, EPA omega-3 oils, vitamin K2, and vitamin D, and needs fatty food with it to be absorbed. Therefore, drinking a glass of tomato juice with no other fat ingestion will not be absorbed (you receive no benefit). The best way, in my opinion, is to eat pizza with cheese (fat soluble) and tomatoes cooked (marinara) on it. Besides, it's fun to eat, and everyone likes pizza!

Twenty-Two

THE SECRETS OF THE PERIPHERAL VASCULAR SYSTEM

The peripheral vascular system involves the veins and arteries in our arms and legs. Although these extremities are most significantly affected by aging and atherosclerosis, there are other considerations. The basic rule is that the farther you get from the heart, the worse the blood vessels can be effected, and this is no exception.

Peripheral vascular disease, I think, deserves this separate chapter, even though it is part and parcel of cardiovascular diseases because it is not well understood or appreciated. It involves the arterial and venous systems into and out of our arms and legs, so let's review its anatomy in order to better understand this condition.

The aorta, which leaves the heart, distributes blood throughout the rest of the body, whether it is to the kidneys, liver, gastrointestinal tract, or legs. The aorta bifurcates or splits in the lower abdomen into the femoral arteries that carry the blood into our legs and then return the blood to the heart and lungs for more oxygen via the femoral veins and inferior vena cava. The arterial blood supply to our arms is carried by the subclavian arteries, but they are seldom affected by serious diseases. Therefore, the femoral arterial and femoral venal diseases make up most of the peripheral vascular diseases that I discuss.

The same risk factors for femoral arterial disease in our legs are the same that we see with coronary disease, such as hypertension, elevated cholesterol and triglyceride levels, and diabetes mellitus. Generically speaking, these patients are called arteriopaths, which means that if there is arterial disease anywhere in their body, it is everywhere. It can result in clogging of our arteries in our legs and causes symptoms of intermittent claudicating, which manifests as pain in the legs with walking that gets better with rest.

Once a diagnosis is made with specialized x-rays such as an MRA (magnetic resonance angiogram), treatment would include an aggressive approach in correcting all the risk factors until they are normalized, along with prescribing vasodilators like Pletal and blood thinners like aspirin and Plavix. At times, especially in severe cases, surgery may be necessary, but always as a last resort.

Our nutrient secret includes arginine, an amino acid, which is also a vasodilator (dilates blood vessels and increases blood flow) of note and should be used in these patients in tandem with the standard medical treatments. Finally, the secret of natural plaque-removing treatments should be implemented like pomegranate, EPA omega-3 oils, omega-7 oils, red-yeast rice, garlic, K2, and olive oil. Arginine works by increasing nitric oxide levels in blood vessels, which dilates them and increases blood flow, and should be an important add-on.

It's important to treat these patients vigorously because gangrene could occur with a resulting amputation, plus the inactivity that it causes results in weight gain and diabetes, and the lack of exercise further exacerbates the cardiac problems. That's called a vicious negative cycle.

You can tell how significant nutrients have become when my university colleagues start a whole new mantra called cardiovascular remodeling. It sounds impressive, but it amounts to a risk-factor reduction; nitric oxide effects on blood vessels; and anti-inflammatory, antioxidant treatments. I have been talking about all these things for five years and have mentioned them in my prior books. Now they play it out with terms like *microvasculature* and *remodeling*. Consider this a victory for the good guys!

It's interesting that the peripheral venous system is *not* affected by the same risk factors that the arterial side is, such as hypertension and diabetes, and it's probably related to lower pressure exposures. Venous disease is mostly related to obesity, pregnancies with vaginal deliveries, drugs that we use like birth control pills (estrogen), or prolonged air travel.

Most of these risk factors share venous compression as a common denominator, but with estrogen, however, it seems that phlebitis results from inflammation of the veins themselves and hyper-coagulation (thick blood) factors. As a result, varicose veins (dilated veins) and edema or swelling of the legs, which goes down in the morning after sleeping, can result. That's called dependent edema. If this condition goes on long enough, however, clots can occur, resulting in thrombophlebitis (blood clots in the legs) with the danger of sudden death from a pulmonary embolism or blood clots into the lungs that break off from the leg clots. There are very few causes of sudden death in humans—strokes, heart attacks, and pulmonary emboli, and this is one of them.

We see this also with prolonged air travel of greater than six hours because people in the cramped seats just don't move their legs. In these scenarios, you should get up every hour and walk around the plane and do calf contractions while sitting in your seat to avoid the clotting.

In obese patients, the situation is worse because the venous back pressure is increased, so the secret here is to lose weight and stay active. Unless you do, the problem will only get worse. Other therapies medically would include wearing support hose, elevating the legs, and taking anticoagulants to avoid a pulmonary embolism, which can cause sudden death. In severe cases, a filter can be placed in the inferior vena cava to prevent emboli moving from the legs into the lungs, which can cause sudden death.

The nutritional secret with peripheral venous disease is that horse chestnut will decrease swelling and also improve the collagen and supportive tissue, thus preventing the problem from getting worse. It may take four to six weeks to work, so be patient. I have not seen any studies yet, but the physiology of pycnogenol also makes sense because of its effect on microcirculation, so the combination of it with horse chestnut could be even more efficacious.

Twenty-Three

THE SECRETS OF OILS

There has been so much new information in regard to oil-treatment protocols that I wanted to include it. These protocols are so all-encompassing in regard to human disease and aging that I thought a separate chapter was necessary. From heart disease to cancer prevention and treatment, oil treatments will surprise you to the point that I recommend them for everyone.

Oils are great for our body's machinery because it would not function long without them. That is why they are such a great secret—because we don't connect oil with our body's metabolic machinery. In the 1970s, Dr. Paul Brunwald at Harvard started an active research program into the omega-3 oils. It followed an epidemiological study that reported that Eskimos (Inuit American Natives) had a low incidence of heart disease, even though they ate a great deal of saturated fats. Later studies reported that their diets, containing high levels of omega-3 oils from the cold-water fish that they ate, were the reason why. Along with this thesis came other sources of the omega-3 oils like flaxseed and krill oils. Finally, along came the omega-7 oils and gamma linoleic acid oils, which, although they may sound the same, are quite different.

The omega-3 oils actually have several mechanisms of action, but the main one is anti-inflammation. The secret in how they do this is quite startling but makes great sense from a body-mechanics point of view. If you had to devise a system that would be turned on by foreign invaders, you would then need a system to turn it off. Otherwise the inflammation would go on forever, and we already know that that is not good (organ scarring with dysfunction and mutations with cancer formation), and that's what the omega-3 oils do. Through proresolution molecules, they actually turn off the whole process, which means that they affect the runoff but do not prevent it like the anti-inflammatory drugs and nutrients would.

The next secret is their ability to decrease cholesterol and LDL (bad cholesterol), but raise the good cholesterol, the HDL. Raising the HDL is not so easy to do, but it also does one additional thing in regard to lipids, which is very important. The omega-3 oils decrease the LpA particle, a very dangerous, tiny LDL molecule that is sometimes called the widow-maker. Again, there are only a few things that will lower this, like niacin, so this ability makes the omega-3 oils a very handy, selective agent.

Finally, in regard to lipids, omega-3 oils help lower the triglyceride level that we see elevated in prediabetics (those with metabolic syndrome or syndrome X). With other inflammatory conditions like colitis (Crohn's disease and ulcerative colitis), omega-3 oils along with folic acid, B12, and wheat grass have become a main player and a must for long-term therapy. The secret with these new nutritional therapies is that most doctors are not even aware of them and will rush patients into the expensive, dangerous drugs without even trying nutrients. Why? Ignorance and ego (I'm important because I use big, bad dangerous drugs.).

Krill oils come from tiny crustaceans found in our seas, which whales eat, and krill oils too are a modest source of omega-3 oils. The secret is krill oils are expensive, and many times the commercial brands do not have much in them. Krill oils appear to have more benefit, however, on the brain than the standard omega-3 oils, so here I would favor them for dementia, strokes, and concussions, which would be good examples. One downside—if you are environmentally concerned, then the overharvesting of krill could affect the balance of nature by harming the fish that eat krill (the whales).

The omega-7 oils sound like the omega-3 oils, but they are not, so don't get them mixed up. Palmitoleic acid (omega-7 oil) from macadamia nuts is most useful with diabetes and serves as an energy mediator (moves calories into the cell) between fat and muscle cells. The omega-7 oils help regulate metabolism, which can help people to lose weight and lower their blood sugars. The omega-7 oils do have a shared benefit with the other lipids, as do the omega-3 oils, but it's the effect on diabetes that should capture your attention. An important secret is that you should not eat the macadamia nuts to get the benefits since the nuts can be toxic (due to palmitic acid) if you eat too many of them.

Most research tells us that nuts daily are also very helpful. People who consume nuts, despite the calories, lose weight and live longer than the patients who do not consume them. It's believed that the monounsaturated oils in nuts are the reason why. As far as which nut is the best, it's the walnut.

There is a great deal of fear in regard to nuts in general, and I think that this is due to the media hype about peanut allergies, but the secret is that we should all be consuming nuts. One secret shown in recent studies is that since we instituted the "don't eat nuts" advice, we now have more nut allergies. One handful daily is prudent. Remember that even if you have a true peanut allergy, you may not be allergic to other nuts. You and your doctor can sort that out. I like that—sort out the nuts!

Active ingredients in flaxseeds are alpha linoleic acid (ALA) and the omega-6 (converted to the omega-3 oils). These oils do all the things that the fish oils will do, but since only about 20 percent is converted, they have an abbreviated effect. Clinical studies show flaxseed consumption to be useful in the treatment of PMS (premenstrual syndrome) and menopause (in women), so the treatment secrets go even beyond inflammation, with hormone intervention. A tiny important secret is that flaxseeds need to be ground up or chewed to have any effect since the seeds otherwise will go straight through you, with no release of the good guys; they are indigestible. Finally, along this hormonal line of thinking, a recent study reported that flaxseed with ALA and phytosterols may help prevent cancer of the prostate.

GLA, or gamma linoleic acid, has found a recent role in pancreatic problems, including cancer of the pancreas. Dr. Ruth Lupu at the Mayo Clinic has done some preliminary work with pancreatic cancer cells and exposing them to GLA. The kill rate is astounding, up to 85–90 percent, and with standard chemotherapy, she is seeing 100 percent cellular kill rates! The secret here is that I treat any of my patients with risks factors for cancer of the pancreas and even pancreatitis with the oil. Incidentally, soy along with curcumin are very useful add-ons also. Oh, if you forgot what the risk factors for pancreatic cancer are, they are increased alcohol intake, diabetes, recurrent bouts of acute pancreatitis (relapsing pancreatitis), and a family history of cancer of the pancreas.

The next secret in the oil arena would be, last but not least, olive oil. The secret active ingredients include the tyrosols (hydoxytyprosol, tyrosol) and oleuropein, whose actions mirror the omega-3 oils, but the end organ effects are different. For example, the extra virgin type (extra virgin is the best) is a great adjunct in treating upper gastrointestinal diseases like esophagus and stomach problems.

A couple ounces three times daily with meals (you can even drink it) is natural, with no side effects. Olive oil also prevents H. pylori, the bacteria that causes stomach ulcers and stomach cancer, from attaching itself to the stomach wall, therefore preventing inflammation. I use this along with DGL, or deglycerolized licorice, and the results are very gratifying, even in patients who have failed with the standard medical regimens. Another secret is the use of cranberry extract along with the above because it too inhibits the H. pylori from its needed attachment to the stomach lining. Don't forget that olive oil also prevents amylin from being converted to toxic peptide aggregate (TPA), which has been linked to diabetes and cancer of the pancreas. Amylin normally helps with insulin function and the lowering of blood sugar.

In summary, I think that you get the message. The secret is to oil your body just like you oil your car, and it too will run better and longer. The analogy is a good one and will hopefully help you remember the importance of oils. Every time you grasp those car keys and start your car, think of your body's engine.

Twenty-Four

THE SECRETS OF SEX

More and more, sex is being recognized as an integral part of our health. Sex-therapy specialists are popping up, and with the advent of low-T (testosterone) syndrome being described and erectile therapies, there is now a new focus.

I titled this chapter "Secrets of Sex" to get your attention, even though "Aphrodisiacs and Their Mechanisms" would be more appropriate. These substances are named after Aphrodite, the mother of Eros (*love*, in Greek), the Greek god with the little bow and arrow; she has been with us for many centuries.

For the Romans, sex was a symbol of prosperity. They felt that duck tongue and bat blood could juice up those sexual feelings. If you look carefully at Roman architecture, you can sense how important it was for them, since they had giant penises everywhere. The Colosseum and their homes were adorned with giant phallic symbols that were meant to symbolize prosperity.

Casanova, another Italian (I'm next—only kidding) from Venice, would eat two dozen oysters before meeting his date, because he claimed that it helped with his sexual prowess. Surprisingly, a recent secret has shown in the laboratory that oysters do in fact increase dopamine pleasure centers in the brain, so he may not have been that wrong with his bragging rights.

The ancients also used foods—or food porn, as they saw them. To them, the fact that some foods looked like genitalia was Mother Nature's way of telling you to eat them for the same reason. Therefore, ipso facto, asparagus, carrots, and bananas were sexual enhancers. For the Aztecs, eating avocados, which looked like giant testicles when hanging on the tree, was the way to enhance their abilities. They actually called them "the testicle trees." We can't leave out the Chinese, however, who revered the rhino horn because it looks like an erection. That's right, an erection.

Evidence for most of this is, of course, lacking, but a more recent secret is that asparagus does contain phytoestrogens that will increase testosterone levels in ten minutes to twenty-four hours, therefore guaranteeing some endurance, except for the "smelly" urine it causes. I can't see the sexual connotation visually, however, unless a bark-looking stem is a turn-on!

More secrets—other natural agents that may have some merit—include arginine, an amino acid that increases penile blood flow much like Viagra and Cialis and therefore supports erections. Pomegranate and pregnenolone increase testosterone levels naturally. Finally, anandamide (which in Sanskrit means *bliss*) stimulates the brain's pleasure messenger center, and it stimulates the same receptors of the brain that marijuana does. Lastly, dark chocolate a vasodilator may help as long as you are not diabetic.

Perhaps the most provocative secret are the scents themselves and their relationship to sex. We've seen animals with their ritual sex dances and how they use scents to find, initiate, and consummate sex. Well, the Smell Center in Chicago also made some very interesting findings. Call me silly, but I was surprised to find out that certain smells were sexual turn-ons for women but were not the same for men. For women, cucumber, licorice, and baby powders were turn-ons, with lavender and pumpkin close seconds, but for men pumpkin, lavender, and donuts were number one. To no one's surprise, it turned out that the men reacted to very low levels of the smells as compared to the women. In fact, it was true that it didn't take much to get the men on the sexual express!

Another secret was the turn-offs for women. That's you, guys, listen up. Cherries, barbecue, and men's cologne were the stop signs of sex for women. In summary, if you are a guy and courting a special lady, don't buy her cherries or wear a cologne and don't take her to a barbecue. Put lots of baby powder on with a hint of cucumber and licorice. Perhaps some cough drops with licorice in them. The secret for the ladies and that special guy are to use a lavender perfume and bring him pumpkin pie with some donuts.

Chocolate candies (dark chocolate) did increase blood flow and endorphins, which would side with the guys as gifts for women. Methylxanthines like theophylline that we use for patients with emphysema and asthma also stimulated the sexual arousal center of the brain.

In summary, the "gigundous" secret for sexual arousal for both men and women is forethought. You need to think about this encounter before you go and adjust your strategies accordingly using this scientific data. I guess it just depends on how much you care about this other person, because just winging it could win the battle but lose the war. Here is some personal advice and a really good secret. A drunken stupor never impresses anyone. How could anyone predicate a long-term relationship on a one-night predatory moment, because even the animal kingdom doesn't abide by those rules? Also, a surefire way to kill an erection is alcohol.

Twenty-Five

THE SECRETS OF GENETICS AND THE ANCIENT GREEKS

When I went to Adelphi, in Greece, even though it was in ruins, I could feel the spirit and energy of the place. The ancient Greeks would go there, on top of a hill overlooking the Corinthian Sea, to have their futures predicted by the oracles. Of course there was a fee, which was identified by the numerous banks that lined the sidewalks going into it. That's right, even back then, banks took your money (some things never change). It was said that many people in high places, including kings and Roman emperors, would not do anything unless cleared first by the oracles.

It's been said that Oedipus consulted the Oracle of Delphi, who told him that he would marry his mother and kill his father, which he, in fact, did. He didn't heed the warnings, however, because he thought that he was stronger than the moment. It's also been said that the historian Herodotus told of King Croesus in Asia Minor, who asked the oracle if he would be a conqueror after invading a particular neighbor. The oracle predicted that if he did, a very powerful nation would fall. Unfortunately, when he did invade, it was his nation that was defeated. How dumb not to ask which one!

I bring this interesting bit of history to you as a preamble to another secret in medicine, which is genetic testing. The parallel is a good one, in that if you know part of the future, will you always make the right decision? In medicine the answer is no, which the ancients told us in their histories, so an explanation is in order.

As of this publication, we have two genetic tests that are relevant to the discussion. The first is the BRCA1 and BRCA2 genes that we see in breast cancer. For women who have a family history of breast cancer (on their mother's side), it is generally recommended that they have this testing done. Roughly 40–80 percent of all breast cancers carry these genes, but not all. If positive, you have a 35–85 percent chance of getting breast cancer, but not 100 percent. Also, if you have both breasts removed to prevent breast cancer, there still is a chance of getting breast cancer because it is physically impossible to remove all the breast tissue.

That's where the Oracle of Delphi comes in, because even with all the data, nothing is 100 percent, and the alternative surgical procedures are very expensive and not without complications (not mentioning the mental component of bilateral breast removal). There is another secret—a medical alternative or choice—that, if you are positive for the gene, get mammograms with an MRI every six months to detect early anything that could be removed if suspicious and take a medication called Arimidex that prevents the likelihood of breast cancer forming. If we have learned anything from the oracles, we have learned that there is nothing in the future with certainty, and when you have to make that decision, be cautious because of the illusion of certainty.

There is another gene of interest called the BRAF gene, and it has also cancer relationships with non-Hodgkin's lymphoma, colon cancer, melanoma, papillary cancer of the thyroid, and both small-cell and adenocarcinoma of the lung. The secret with the BRAF gene is not its prognostic ability, but treatment choices. The genetic foul-up here is a protein called B-Raf that sends signals in cells that impact cell growth. Because of this ability, with faulty mutated genes, its presence can lead to the cancers that were mentioned earlier.

The Oracle of Delphi here would be much more definitive, because she would tell you that if gene positive, take the drug therapy. Zelboraf and Vemurafenib work extremely well, but after a short time, 20–50 percent will become resistant to the drugs, but the remaining tumors won't. Since there is no illusion of certainty here, just the facts, perhaps the oracle wouldn't charge you so much!

My advice to my patients and you alike is a secret that has worked extremely well. There are no banks lining the sidewalk leading to my office, so there is no financial gain to be made. I tell my patients and their families that before I do these genetic tests, they have to make their decisions on what to do if the result is positive. The reason is that if the testing is positive, there is so much mental overlay with stress that any decisions are almost impossible and tainted with emotion. Decisions have to be made before the storm arrives. Once clear on your decision, then go ahead with the testing. However, cancers come back, there will be some form of relief. In my experience, gene testing, like stem cell research, has not helped much in regard to taking care of people but has carried a badge-of-honor mentality that only distorts the decision-making process.

Twenty-Six

The Secrets of a Simple yet Complex Medical Problem—Halitosis (Bad Breath)

It's sometimes the simple things that get us down, and I guess they are too trivial to be deemed important, but if they are affecting you, it is 100 percent. The other thing to remember is that the simple, common things over time can create much worse medical diseases that you would prefer not to have.

The secret with halitosis, or bad breath, is that it can be a real killer in many ways, but because of its impact on social and workplace situations, you should *always* tell someone that he or she has it, because the person cannot smell it. Breathing into your hand and then rebreathing the air will not tell you if you have it.

By far the most common problems causing it are mouth problems. Chronic tooth, gum, tonsil, and sinus infections are the most common causes of bad breath, so generally a dental appointment will be necessary, along with a good exam of the oral cavity and sinuses. A dry mouth due to insufficient saliva can lead to these problems, so the salivary glands need to be checked out, along with a Sjogren's syndrome work-up that can do the same thing (dry mouth, dry eyes, and arthritis). Here seeing an ENT specialist, along with blood immune tests for Sjogren's, should be done.

Chronic lung problems like chronic bronchitis with increased phlegm may do the same thing, but here the sputum by history is purulent (yellow-green) and has an odor. Liver diseases can give off sulfur; kidney disease can give off ammonia; and H. pylori, the bacteria that cause stomach ulcers and stomach cancer, may cause halitosis also. The esophagus, with outpouchings called diverticula, or a Zenker's diverticulum because of undigested food in them can also cause bad breath. In addition, low-acid stomach conditions like pernicious anemia (B12 deficiency) and achlorhydria can do the same.

An important secret is to hunt down the cause because most times you will find it and, with treatment, get rid of it. Incidentally, pernicious anemia is a pre-cancerous stomach condition, so if that is the cause, a yearly upper endoscopy may be in order to diagnose a stomach cancer early.

Supportive therapies include drinking more water, chewing sugarless gum, and using artificial saliva. Brushing with an electric toothbrush twice daily with a fluoride toothpaste along with flossing with fluorinated floss will help immensely. Of course, finding the root cause, and its treatment is fundamentally the key. Probiotics (good bacteria) and tongue scrapings, especially of the posterior tongue area, may help, but the specific research is lacking. What can it hurt? Mouthwashes, even Listerine, may help for up to one to two hours, but at best it's a temporary cure.

As you can see, the secret for such a seemingly trivial problem's work-up can be extensive. I can't stress enough, however, how important the work-up is, because a cancer may be lingering in the shadows. One thing that they try to teach us in medical school is to never dismiss a trivial problem that could be a catastrophe down the road. You just need the training to know the difference. Besides the obvious social consequences that it creates, bad breath may jeopardize a workplace opportunity.

Twenty-Seven

The Secrets of Acetylcysteine in Treating Lung Disease and Other Uses

The lungs for many years have been left behind in regard to nutrient therapies, but with newer discoveries, like free radicals in the lungs and oxidative damage from inflammation and exercising, new nutritional frontiers have been opened up. We now have a drug, Daliresp that only treats inflammation of the lung—a sign that the standard practice of medicine is waking up to these basic concepts. We discussed this earlier, but let's take a closer look.

One way of looking at your body is to consider it a bank. Yes, a bank that saves and stores important things like money—money that you can use in the future for that rainy day. The secret here is instead of storing money, the body stores antioxidants. During the course of any day, your body goes through many oxidative metabolic processes, requiring oxygen and creating these free radicals that are atoms with a missing outer-ring electron. Unless neutralized by electron donors (antioxidants), free radicals can wreak havoc with cellular function and lead to inflammation and DNA mutations with cancer over time.

Now, if your body's bank were full of antioxidants, then both short- and long-term problems could theoretically be preempted and hopefully avoided. The secret here is to save, like banks do, enough antioxidants to do this very thing. The antioxidants in this savings account would come from two sources.

One exogenous source, from outside your body, would be vitamins, minerals, and herbs that you consume and take in. The other source is endogenous, what your body makes. One of the major endogenous sources for these electrons is glutathione, which is made in the liver. Just as a corollary to all this, studies have confirmed that people with the highest antioxidant levels live longer than those with lower levels. What I want to do now is review a way to increase the endogenous glutathione, which directly helps our lungs to fight off the free radicals.

N-acetyl cysteine (not cystine), or NAC, is an amino acid derivative that first made its prominence as a respiratory inhalant. Chemically, it is a modified variant of the sulfur-containing cysteine, and, like I said, it made its first appearance as a mucolytic agent (breaks down mucous) in severe respiratory problems like with COPD (emphysema, chronic obstructive lung disease) and cystic fibrosis. Very early in its development, it was discovered to increase the liver's production of glutathione and was used to treat Tylenol overdoses.

The reason for this was that Tylenol overwhelmed the liver's capacity to make glutathione and destroyed the liver two to three days later, but the NAC, however, very quickly restored the liver level back to normal. NAC was also found to affect certain genes, with the first being the signaling genes of inflammation, which were mostly derived from the research that was being done on the influenza virus.

The influenza virus, once in our body, results in a "storm" release of pro-inflammates (chemicals of inflammation), which was inhibited by NAC along with suppressing the "master signal" molecule NFkB or nuclear factor kappa beta. This NFkB is a transcriptor that hooks onto the DNA, telling it what to do in regard to cell division. In addition, NAC regulates the gene for COX-2—the enzyme that produces pain and swelling (inflammation), which many medications do, like the COX-2 inhibitors such as Arthrotec and Voltaren. We use these drugs frequently in the treatment of arthritis for this reason. The ability of the NAC to go into the cell itself also protects the DNA, which is always a good idea.

A very important secret that most people and many doctors are not aware of is that influenza is a very serious problem, but because it comes around every year and we do have vaccinations, we all tend to dismiss it and take it for granted. We shouldn't, because the virus causes cell death to the lining cells of our lungs, which can lead to a fatal pneumonia or permanent lung damage. When looking at the virus under the microscope, scientists describe what the virus does to cells as "cell boiling." Well, NAC negates this boiling process almost immediately, and if given prophylactically, it doesn't happen at all. That means that if you are at risk for influenza—for example, if you are elderly, immunally compromised, or have influenza—take the NAC 600–1,200 mg per day.

The next step or secret is not a giant one, but an appropriate one, and it affects many millions of people every day. I'm talking about COPD, or chronic obstructive lung disease, which we find in smokers; in workers in certain industries such as coal, silicon, and asbestos; in those with chronic bronchitis and long-standing asthma; and in anyone who has a long-term lung problem like sarcoid.

With COPD, one study found that 600 mg/day of NAC doubled the rate of bacterial eradication from the study participants' lungs. The reason is the profound NAC down-regulating inflammatory cytokines and NFkB responses. One unique disease, idiopathic pulmonary fibrosis (IPF), has extreme cellular inflammatory reaction levels, but cellular levels in the lungs of the NAC patients are almost zero. Oral and aerosolized medications of NAC in these patients improve lung function by three times and give them more hope.

A unique twist and new secret has to do with lung function and exercise. Since strenuous exercise increases metabolic function, it also creates more free radicals. Tissue levels, especially in the lungs, of the inflammatory cytokines (inflammatory chemicals) like tumor necrosis factor (TNF) go up dramatically and, if not neutralized, can cause lung damage (that burning feeling in your lungs that you experience with intense exercise). That's right—you inadvertently damage your lungs with intensive exercise. It's been reported that taking NAC prior to exercise increases endurance by 25 percent and dramatically decreases the oxidative proteins created with the exercise. Here you are looking at about 1,800–2,000 mg/day.

For me, the greatest secret relates to NAC and diabetes mellitus. Insulin resistance is a gigantic problem with adult diabetes, which means that these diabetics make plenty of insulin but it doesn't work. As our research gets better and a clearer picture evolves, it seems to directly relate to oxidation and free radicals. The free radicals impair the insulin receptors that cause blood sugars to rise along with the development of advanced glycation end products (AGEs) that attach themselves to the proteins, making them inactive, including the cellular DNA. NAC reverses many of these influences and also interrupts the evil empire of high fructose corn syrup (HFCS). HFCS, when ingested, immediately goes to the liver and does not require insulin, which makes it different than sugar. Blood pressures and blood sugars go up, uric acid becomes elevated (gout), along with increased triglycerides, which are all reversed with NAC. In polycystic ovarian disease, where there are hormonal imbalances and blood sugar elevations, NAC (1,200–1,600 mg/day) and arginine will normalize them.

I guess that it won't surprise you that there are also cancer secrets with NAC, involving mainly the skin, lung, stomach, and colon. In stomach cancers it induces apoptosis (cell suicide) and stops DNA synthesis therefore stopping cancer cell multiplication. It also inhibits NFkB in melanotic cancers, preventing expressions of the signaling proteins that are required for cancer growth. Another rather unique ability of NAC is to inactivate and destroy c-Src, a chemical control molecule that allows cancers to grow. Finally, there are clinical studies showing that NAC can prevent colon polyps (40 percent) and cancer along with reducing the risks of lung cancer with smokers. In these patients, there was a decrease in precancerous cells and damaged DNA markers. It's becoming clear that patients who are at risk for these cancers should be on NAC. Now that's a secret!

The last but not least effect is on H. pylori, the bacteria that cause stomach ulcers and gastric cancer. There are two secrets, with the first being that NAC reduces inflammation through gene expression, reducing the hydrogen peroxide production that is induced by the bacteria. Second, it inhibits the actual growth of the bacteria. To do this, 600–1,200 mg/day is recommended.

In summary, NAC, or N-acetyl cysteine, needs to be a serious consideration for patients who are at risk or have lung disease, diabetes, Tylenol toxicity, influenza, cancer, and H. pylori. Not a bad collection of secrets, but a better understanding of the medical problems will help mandate its importance. If prevention is your game, and it should be, NAC has to be a major player. It's not a panacea, I grant you by any stretch, but within its proper context, it's a Babe Ruth home run!

Twenty-Eight

WHAT'S HAPPENING TODAY

As you have probably figured out already, most of this information is not truly a secret, since no one, at least deliberately, has been hiding a known fact. The problem is a faulty information system. There is a "grand canyon" separation between research and the consumers, with their doctors as the intermediary. For me, this is where the real secret lies.

Doctors are not keeping up, whether intentionally or unintentionally, so the patient is being left behind. Ironically, when it comes to nutrient or alternative therapies, most physicians are, for the most part, not interested, which again puts patients on the short end of this stick. I would guess that patients know more about nutrient therapies than most doctors, and that is a sad secret and commentary. Instead of acknowledging and accepting this lack of knowledge, the medical profession, however, in general has put a pox on it.

For me, a standard practicing physician who went through a standard university teaching program, I am both surprised and disappointed in my fellow physicians. I truly think that the reason why they are so complacent is that they are totally distracted by a profession in change and are only trying to survive as their reimbursements go down and down.

For example, for endoscopic procedures for which I got paid $600–$700 dollars fifteen years ago, I now receive $200. For an EKG fifteen years ago, I was paid $75 dollars, but now it's $25. Of course, this is in the framework of my expenses going up every year, along with my medical malpractice insurance (remember those bloodthirsty attorneys).

We as physicians, when we went to meetings, used to discuss interesting cases, but now the conversation is only about surviving and the government and insurance companies and what they are doing to us. You as a patient ask for medical care, and we deliver it (the best in the world, by the way), and then the government (Medicare) and the insurance companies do everything, from delays to audits, and then don't pay us under the heading of "not indicated." They hire other companies to give us guidelines, as if we don't know how to take care of you, when in fact these companies are nothing more than clinical guidelines to save them money and serve as a template for more payment rejections.

The Mayo Clinic, by the way, has on several occasions reviewed those guidelines and reported that they don't work! The end result of all this—and it's only a guess—is that my fellow physicians are in the struggle for their life, and everyone, including their own organizations like the AMA, has sold them out. So why should they get involved in something new (prescribing nutrient supplements) that's going to cost them money to learn, and they won't be reimbursed by the third-party payers?

The secret here is that it is today's reality and is currently affecting you in a death spiral that will end in a very different world. Medicine as you know it will be no more and will be broken down into two levels of care: one, a government-controlled one, even mandating through insurance carriers; and the other a cash business, a boutique-type model that you can choose if you want to spend the money. The patients who are able to take advantage of the latter model will have immediate access to the best doctors, facilities, and testing. The others won't and will have to wait.

How do I know this? Because I've seen the first system up close and personal in Canada and all through Europe. Here's the kicker. Our government wants the first form, while, yes, our elected politicians will make sure that they have the latter form. This is beginning to sound like a sermon, and for that I must apologize, but all these secrets must be discussed, especially when they are affecting you.

It's my hope that in reading this book and assessing your own situation, you will get involved and, along with your doctors, not their organizations, will stop the bleeding before it's too late. I have given you new concepts on which to base your nutrient regimens and have also given them some legitimacy and understanding. Make no mistake about it, nutrients are chemicals that affect our metabolic engines just like medications and can have great benefit or great harm, so use them judiciously.

As you would guess, I take many of them, but in the context of my medical profile, and I take medications that I am sure give me the stamina, endurance, and positive attitude to do what I do. How do I know? When I stop them for just a few days, I notice the difference, and I don't like the feeling!

There are also other new frontiers in medicine, such as immunotherapy for cancer prevention and treatment and anti-inflammatory effects for immune diseases, and they too are becoming inundated with nutrient therapies. That tells me how important they are, along with the whole new field of antiaging and the ability to preempt death.

Nutrients really give us ammunition to be proactive in our health, along with sorting out risk factors, instead of waiting for something to happen, which could be a fatal heart attack. You don't get a second chance here. I would hope that nutrition becomes part of your life—without the myths that fill our society today. Organic, free-range, and gluten-free diets are some of the distractions that have no basis and need to be avoided. Focus your time, energy, and money where it belongs—on your own and your family's survival!

About the Author

David L. Vastola, DO, is AMA board certified in internal medicine and gastroenterology. He has been an adjunct professor in the Palm Beach Atlantic University School of Pharmacy (nutritional studies) for thirteen years.

He is the former chief of gastroenterology at Deaconess Hospital Buffalo and assistant professor of medicine and pharmacy at the State University of New York at Buffalo. Prior to that he was an attending at Buffalo Children's Hospital and a special attending in Niagara Falls Hospitals and at the Seneca Indian reservation regarding comprehensive GI problems. After that, Dr. Vastola practiced private medicine for thirty-five years in south Florida in the field of internal medicine and gastroenterology. Also, he was on live radio for twenty years for two hours every week and did segments for eight years on his local Fox-TV station's ten o'clock news program, five days a week. Finally, he currently serves as adjunct professor of medicine in the Gregory School of Pharmacy, Palm Beach Atlantic University, where he has been for twelve years, and is currently teaching nutrition studies.

Dr. Vastola has published research in the *Journal of Chest Surgery* and held a one-year tenure on the medical admissions committee at the State University of New York at Buffalo. He was a board member of the Juvenile Diabetic Association for three years in Palm Beach County, and was accepted for but declined both an advanced GI immunity fellowship at the Mayo Clinic and a one-year fellowship of advance endoscopy at Yale University.

Made in the USA
Columbia, SC
16 March 2019